Children in the New Millennium

Environmental Impact on Health

UNEP unicef WHO

Children in the New Millennium:
Environmental Impact on Health

Library of Congress Cataloguing in Publication Data

Children in the New Millennium:
Environmental Impact on Health

UNEP, UNICEF & WHO – 2002
Endnotes
Includes index

ISBN: 92-807-2065-1

1. Environment 2. Children 3. Health
4. Sustainable Development

Online version can be found at
www.unep.org, www.unicef.org and www.who.int

Printed on recycled paper in the Republic of Malta

Table of Contents

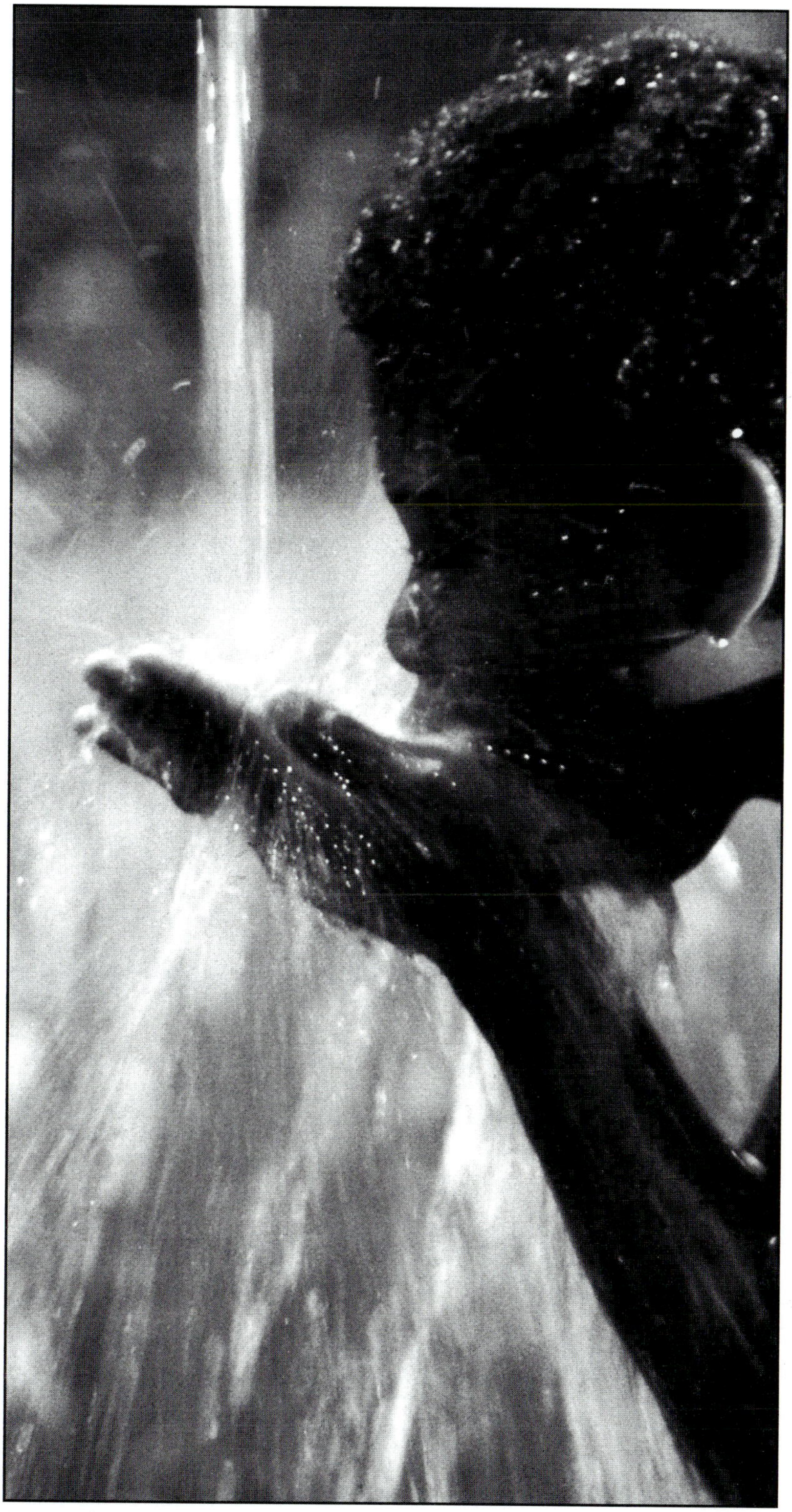

A healthy future for our children will be ensured only through safeguarding the environment.

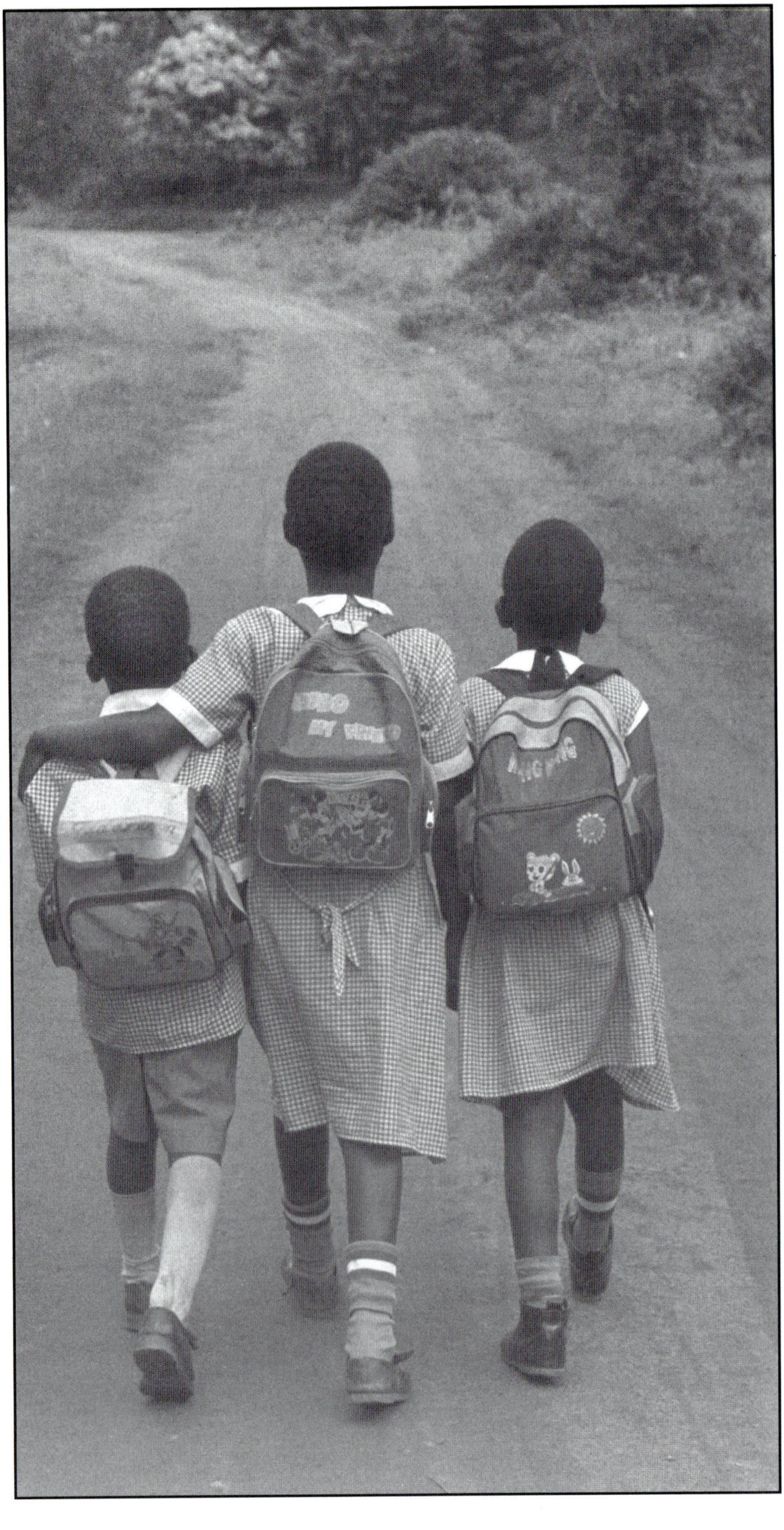

Over the past ten years, great strides have been made to safeguard the health and well-being of our children.

Foreword

Over the past ten years, great strides have been made to safeguard the health and well-being of our children. Millions of young lives have been saved as a result of increased immunization coverage and expanded basic social services, including primary health care, children's and women's nutrition programmes, and adequate water supply and sanitation. More children than ever are in school and important treaties and policies have been concluded or adopted by the international community and national governments to strengthen environmental protection measures and protect children from exploitation.

Yet for all the advances made, children everywhere continue to suffer the consequences of environmental degradation. Collapsing ecosystems leave them less able to realize their rights and sustain their basic needs: clean food, air and water. Children are often the canaries in the coal mines. Their health is a key barometer of the long-term effects of the decisions and activities of adults.

One decade ago, the precursor to this publication *Children and the Environment,* jointly published by the United Nations Environment Programme (UNEP) and the United Nations

Children's Fund (UNICEF), warned its readers that, "environmental degradation is killing children." Today, that warning echoes even louder.

Children are exposed to a series of environmental threats to their health, physical and mental development – even their survival. Preliminary estimates suggest that up to one-third of the global burden of disease can be attributed to negative environmental indicators, such as polluted water and air. The good news is that morbidity and mortality due to unhealthy environmental conditions are largely preventable by taking decisive action and finding innovative, healthy, cost-effective and sustainable ways to develop and improve our livelihoods.

As this book outlines, prevention is the only sustainable solution: a healthy future for our children will be ensured only through safeguarding the environment. By illustrating the link between the environment and the well-being of our children, *Children in the New Millennium* intends to raise awareness and deepen our understanding of environmental health issues. Providing an informed basis for action and practical recommendations at different levels, the three United Nations agencies involved with the production of *Children in the New Millennium* hope to inspire everyone who cares about children to take decisive action that will improve both their health and that of the environment.

As this book goes to press, the international community is engaged in two related intergovernmental processes to review the progress made since the 1990 World Summit for Children and the 1992 United Nations Conference on Environment and Development (the "Earth Summit"). The reviews will culminate at the Special Session of the United Nations General Assembly on Children in May 2002 and the World Summit on Sustainable Development in August 2002. Taking advantage of these opportunities, this book highlights in a timely manner the mutually reinforcing goals of realising children's rights and managing environmental challenges of the 21st century.

Children's environmental health issues have been recognized in many international agreements and declarations over the past decade. The challenge before us now is to translate the words of declarations into actions and emerge ten years from now having addressed the linkages between children's health and the environment in a meaningful and measurable way. In ten years the children on this planet should be healthier and happier as a result of the decisions and actions we all take today.

We are presently witnessing an unprecedented pace of development in the world alongside overwhelming social, economic and environmental transformations. In this era of rapid change, it is imperative that we rally the will and the imagination of us all to seize upon every opportunity to preserve the health of our environment and create a better future for our children.

A decade ago UNEP and UNICEF affirmed that, "we owe our children a planet fit to live on and capable of sustaining the future." We have the opportunity and the responsibility to fulfil this pledge. UNEP, UNICEF and the World Health Organization (WHO) are fully committed within their spheres, and together, to foster collaboration among UN agencies, governments and civil society to place children's environmental health interests at the forefront of our agendas.

Klaus Töpfer
Executive Director
UNEP

Carol Bellamy
Executive Director
UNICEF

Gro Harlem Brundtland
Director General
WHO

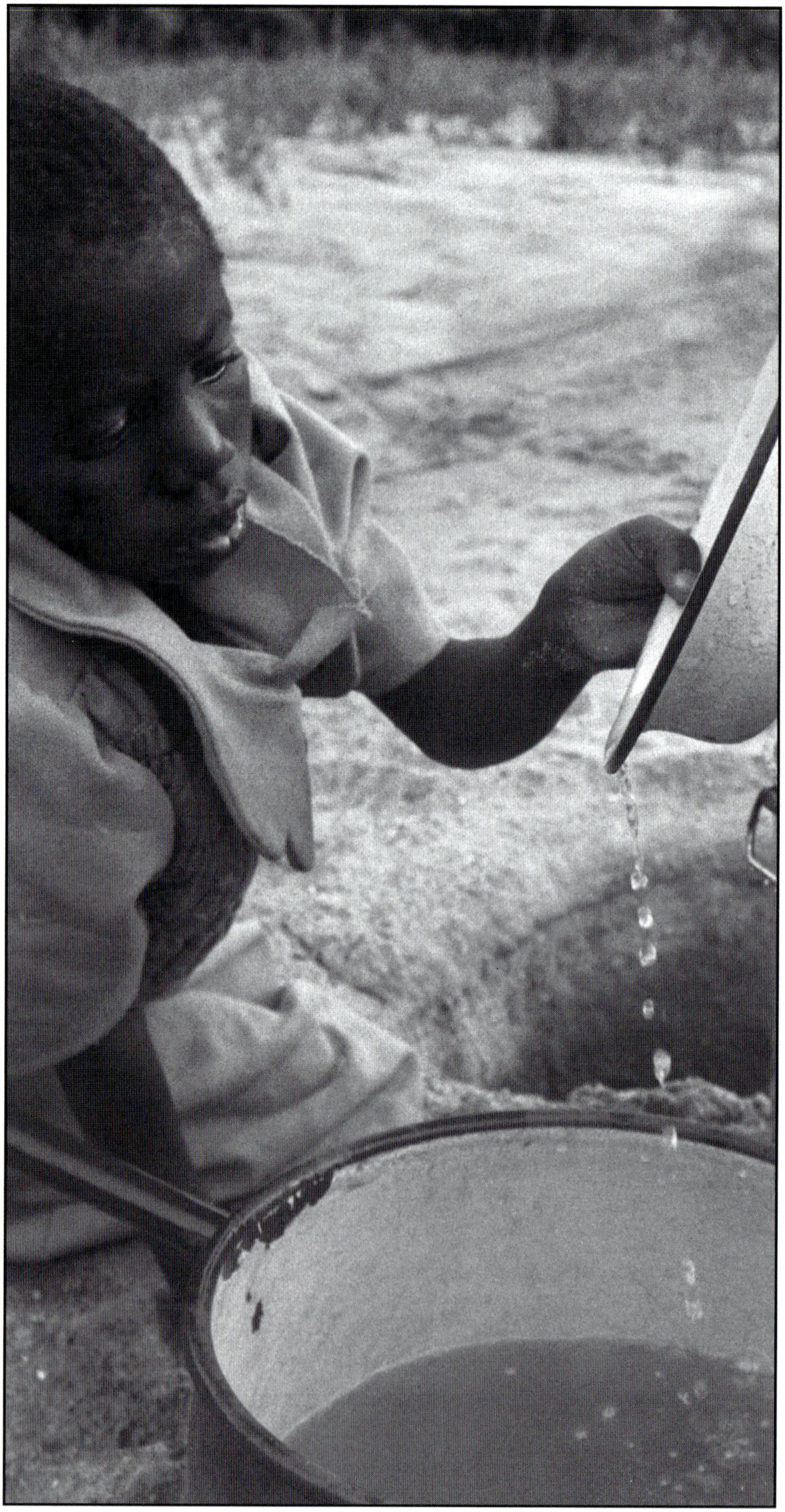

Environmental quality is one of the key factors in determining whether a child survives the first years of life.

Acknowledgements

This booklet is the result of close collaboration between three agencies of the United Nations system: the Environment Programme (UNEP), the United Nations Children's Fund (UNICEF) and the World Health Organization (WHO). Many colleagues in the three organizations rendered helpful advice and encouragement during the development of this booklet. Particular thanks go to the following individuals who provided valuable input:

Mansoor Ali (UNICEF), Adnan Amin (UNEP), Monika Blössner (WHO), Lizette Burgers (UNICEF), Carlos Corvalan (WHO), Carlos Dora (WHO), Hiremagalur Gopalan (UNEP), Jose Hueb (WHO), Eva Jespersen (UNICEF), Theresa Kilbane (UNICEF), Ken Legins (UNICEF), TV Luong (UNICEF), Anna-Maria Mooijman (UNICEF), Richard Morgan (UNICEF), Theodore Oben (UNEP), Annette Pruess (WHO), Eva Rehfuess (WHO), Dorothy Rozga (UNICEF), Dietrich Schwela (WHO), James Sniffen (UNEP), Hans Spruijt (UNICEF) and Vanessa Tobin (UNICEF).

In addition to the above, the following external experts reviewed the draft and made very useful contributions:

Dr. Lilian Corra (Chair, Asociacion Argentina de Medicos por el Medio Ambiente, Vice-President, International Society of Doctors for the Environment, Coordinating Committee Member, International Research and Information Network on Children's Health, Environment and Safety); Dr. Tewolde Berhan Gebre Egziabher (General Manager, Environmental Protection Authority, Ethiopia); Dr. Janusz Haluska (Head, Department of Health and Environment Jagiellonian University, Krakow, Poland); Dr. Peter van den Hazel, (Founder and International Coordinator, International Research and Information Network on Children's Health, Environment and Safety, Chairman, Dutch Association of Environmental Medicine, Vice-President Europe, International Society of Doctors for the Environment); Karen Hopfl-Harris, (Legislative Director, Environment and Health Programs, Physicians for Social Responsibility, Washington D.C., USA); Dr. Irma R. Makalinao (Associate Professor, Department of Pharmacology and Toxicology, University of the Philippines College of Medicine); Dr. Sherif M. Shawky (Associate Professor, Environmental Chemistry and Biology, Environmental Health Department, Alexandria University, High Institute of Public Health, Egypt); and Susan T. West (Director, Environment and Health Programs, Physicians for Social Responsibility, Washington D.C., USA).

The book was developed by Maaike Jansen of UNEP, Jingjing Qian of UNICEF and environmental consultant Marisha Wojciechowska-Shibuya, with substantive contributions from Jenny Pronczuk of WHO. Patricia Lone and Christine Dinsmore edited the book. Gillian Haggerty produced the layout and oversaw the printing.

1 The Context

Introduction

Children embody our dreams and our hopes for the future. They also inherit our legacies, including the consequences of how we treat the natural environment. At the dawn of the 21st century, nearly 11 million children still die every year of readily preventable causes[1], the equivalent of some 29,000 children dying every single day. Environmental quality is one of the key factors in determining whether a child survives the first years of life, and strongly influences the child's subsequent physical and mental development[2].

Excessive and wasteful consumption, social inequities and inefficient resource use perpetuate a vicious cycle of pollution and resource degradation that contribute to poverty and the erosion of livelihoods. These conditions severely harm adults and children, particularly those living in ecologically vulnerable areas.

Children are at greater risk from environmental hazards because of their physical size, immature organs, metabolic rate, behaviour, natural curiosity and lack of knowledge. With the current trend of environmental degradation, children have fewer and

[1] *All endnotes are at the back of the book, beginning on page 119.*

With proper support, children can acquire useful knowledge from participating in environmental activities and can contribute in a unique manner, with energy and vision, to finding solutions.

fewer places to hide. They can even be exposed to harmful environmental hazards before birth.

On the other hand, children are also dynamic and powerful forces for environmental protection. They show a natural interest in nature and are often passionate about the preservation of their planet. With proper support, children can acquire useful knowledge from participating in environmental activities and can contribute in a unique manner, with energy and vision, to finding solutions.

The link between children and the environment has been recognized in numerous international declarations and agreements over the past decade (see box 1). This booklet offers a succinct overview of environmental issues affecting the health, development and well-being of children and presents the state of knowledge in this field, conceding that significant gaps exist in the information and data available. For people working at the international, national, local and household levels with children, health and/or environmental issues, this document encourages inter-disciplinary thinking and suggests concrete recommendations for action.

Progress Made Since the World Summit for Children and the United Nations Conference on Environment and Development

Outcomes from two global conferences have explicitly established the linkages between children and the environment. At the 1990 World Summit for Children, leaders adopted a World Declaration and Plan of Action, recognising that "children have the greatest stake in the preservation of the environment and its judicious management for sustainable development as their survival and development depends on it."[3] Subsequently, the 1992 United Nations Conference on Environment and Development (UNCED, also known as "The Earth Summit") adopted the Rio Declaration and Agenda 21, a world action plan for sustainable development, which includes a chapter on children and youth.

Governments made a series of commitments at UNCED, which encompass the goals of the World Summit for Children.

It is useful to provide an overview of where we stand a decade later with respect to the commitments made at these two international conferences in terms of protecting our children and safeguarding the environment.

Since the World Summit for Children

A series of goals were adopted at the World Summit for Children, which, if achieved, would fulfil the rights enshrined in the Convention on the Rights of the Child. During the 1990s, progress was made towards fulfilling these goals. Millions of young lives have been saved as a result of increased immunization coverage and expanded basic social services, including primary health care, children's and women's nutrition programmes and clean water supply and adequate sanitation. At the global level, the international community has adopted numerous critically important treaties and policies to protect children from exploitation.

Over 60 countries have achieved the Summit goal of a one third reduction in mortality among children under the age of five; in over 100 countries, under-five deaths were cut by one fifth during the decade[4] (see figure 1). Most notably, the deaths of young children from diarrhoeal diseases – one of the leading causes of the under-five mortality rate – were reduced by 50 per cent, saving more than a million lives every year[5].

Yet in spite of these advances, many of the promises for children made at the World Summit and subsequent international conferences of the past decade remain unfulfilled and the lives of countless children and their families continue to be blighted. In addition to the nearly 11 million children dying from readily preventable causes each year, an estimated 150 million children in the developing world are malnourished[6]. Over 120 million are still out of school, 53 per cent of them girls[7]. Unprecedented incidences of civil wars and ethnic conflicts marked the last decade, with perhaps more children losing their lives than ever before.

Box 1: Links Between Children and the Environment in Selected International Agreements

Convention on the Rights of the Child (1989): "To combat disease and malnutrition, including within the framework of primary health care, through, *inter alia*, the application of readily available technology and through the provision of adequate nutritious foods and clean drinking-water, taking into consideration the dangers and risks of environmental pollution" *and* "States Parties agree that the education of the child shall be directed to: … the development of respect for the natural environment."

Plan of Action for Implementing the World Declaration on the Survival, Protection and Development of Children in the 1990s: "… to improve the environment by combating disease and malnutrition and promoting education. These contribute to lowering death rates as well as birth rates, improved social services, better use of natural resources and, ultimately, to the breaking of the vicious cycle of poverty and environmental degradation."

Agenda 21 (1992): "The health of children is affected more severely than other population groups by malnutrition and adverse environmental factors." *and*, "Children not only will inherit the responsibility of looking after the Earth, but in many developing countries they comprise nearly half the population…. Children in both developing and industrialized countries are highly vulnerable to the effects of environmental degradation… The specific interests of children need to be taken fully into account in the participatory process on environment and development."

The Habitat Agenda (1996): "The needs of children and youth, particularly with regard to their living environment, have to be taken fully into account."

Declaration of the Environment Leaders of the Eight on Children's Environmental Health (1997): "We acknowledge that, throughout the world, children face significant threats to health from an array of environmental hazards. The protection of human health remains a fundamental objective of environmental policies to achieve sustainable development. We increasingly understand that the health and well-being of our families depend upon a clean and healthy environment. Nowhere is this more true than in the case of children, who are particularly vulnerable to pollution… We affirm that prevention of exposure is the single most effective means of protecting children against environmental threats."

G8 Environment Ministers Communiqué (2001): "We are determined to develop policies and implement actions to provide children with a safe environment, including during prenatal and postnatal development, towards the highest attainable level of health." *and* "We recognize that poverty and insufficient protection from environmental threats are often found in tandem. We will work together to address the most serious environmental health threats, including microbiological and chemical contaminants in drinking water, air pollution that exacerbates illness and death from asthma and other respiratory problems, polluted water, toxic substances and pesticides."

The Berlin Commitment for Children of Europe and Central Asia (2001): "Protect all children, irrespective of the social and economic conditions they live in from environmental threats; create child-respecting urban and rural environments which enable all children to have access to a range of play and informal learning opportunities both at home and within their local communities."

Figure 1: Under-five mortality rate, change over period 1990-2000

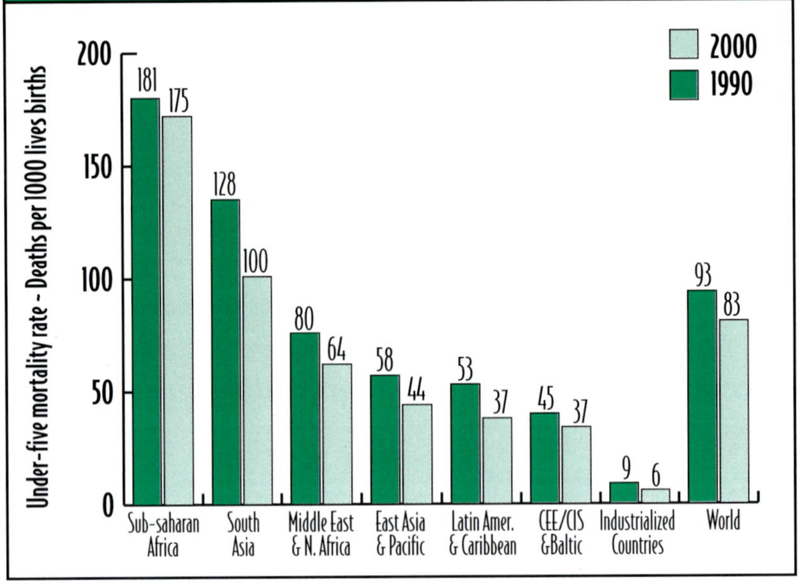

Source: United Nations Children's Fund (UNICEF), Progress since the World Summit for Children: A Statistical Review, page 3, UNICEF, New York, September 2001; and UNICEF, The State of the World's Children 2002, table 8, UNICEF, New York, 2002.

HIV/AIDS is reaching catastrophic levels, particularly in sub-Saharan Africa, robbing millions of children of their parents, schoolteachers and village nurses. In addition, far too many children continue to live without clean drinking water and adequate sanitation.

During the 1990s, the global community recognized children's right to a clean, healthy environment. At the 1992 United Nations Conference on Environment and Development, UNICEF proclaimed "we must preserve our planet in order to nurture our children; equally, we must nurture our children if we are to preserve our planet."[8] At the 2000 United Nations Millennium Summit, the international community reinforced this commitment with its adoption of the Millennium Declaration. Among the resolutions was the goal to halve the proportion of people living in poverty and those suffering from hunger and lack of safe drinking water by 2015.

The Millennium Declaration's principle is also echoed in the Say Yes Campaign of the Global Movement for Children (see box

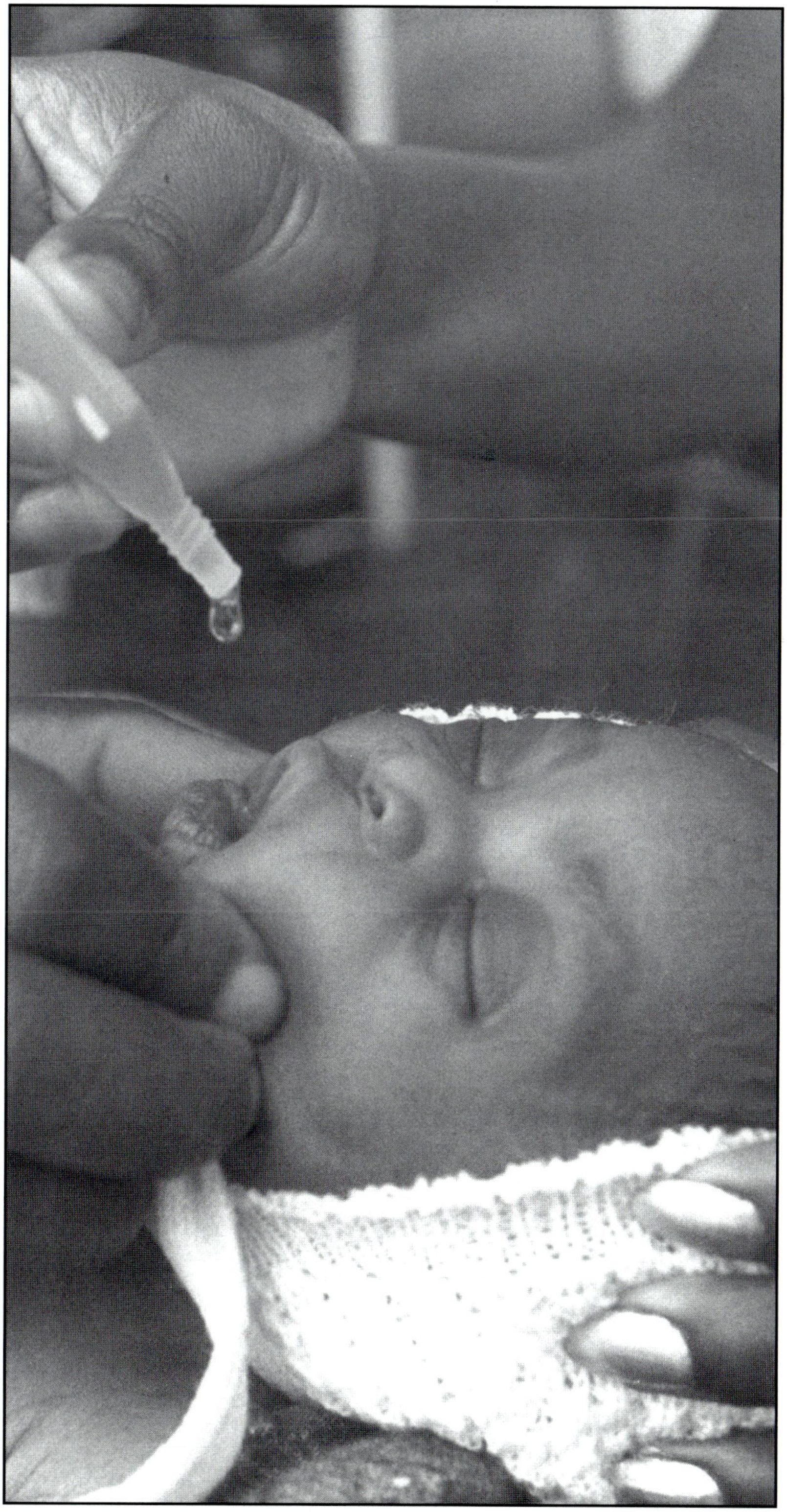

Among the goals of Millennium Declaration was to halve the proportion of people living in poverty and those suffering from hunger and lack of safe drinking water by 2015.

2), championed by Nelson Mandela and Graça Machel, which calls for people throughout the world to take action and protect the rights of children, including protecting the earth for children.

The Special Session on Children of the United Nations General Assembly in May 2002 will serve to review the progress achieved in the last decade. It will also provide an opportunity for world leaders to reaffirm their obligation to safeguard the rights of all children through enhanced national action and international cooperation to make the world fit for children.

Box 2: Say Yes for Children

As this book goes to press, over 44 million women, men and children have pledged to "Say Yes for Children" in a world-wide campaign and have rallied behind ten overarching principles that seek to improve and protect the lives of children. One of these principles relates to environmental protection and has received wide support from the people who made their pledges. The world leaders attending the Special Session on Children will formally adopt these principles together with a series of supporting actions to make a world safe for children. The ten principles are:

- Leave no child out
- Put children first
- Care for every child
- Fight HIV/AIDS
- Stop harming and exploiting children
- Listen to children
- Educate every child
- Protect children from war
- Protect the earth for children
- Fight poverty: invest in children

Source: Global Movement for Children (http://www.gmfc.org/en)

Since UNCED

The concept of sustainable development adopted at UNCED provides an over-arching policy framework within which the international community addresses the environmental, social and economic dimensions of development. From the environmental dimension, notable progress has been made on several fronts since 1992, from the negotiation and implementation of a remarkable number of multilateral environmental agreements, to the widespread efforts on the local level to implement the recommendations of Agenda 21. Furthermore, the realization that environmental challenges need to be addressed in all their complexity is increasingly entering the mainstream. This is reflected, for example, in the attention accorded environmental issues in national and local political processes; in the vibrancy of the non-governmental sector; in the unprecedented media coverage devoted to environmental degradation and its impacts; and in the innovations and initiatives being undertaken by the private sector in response to changing consumer attitudes.

Nonetheless, in the context of the gravity and urgency of the environmental challenges facing the international community, the relatively gradual improvements achieved since UNCED are widely regarded as insufficient to meet the commitments made at that time.

Global environmental degradation continues at an alarming rate, fuelled by social and economic problems such as pervasive poverty, unsustainable production and consumption patterns, inequity in distribution of wealth, unequal access to resources, uneven impacts of globalization and the debt burden. Numerous studies offer compelling evidence of the immensity of the environmental challenges facing us. For example, it has become increasingly evident that:

- The world water cycle will be unable to cope with demands in the coming decades, and if present trends continue two out of three people will live in water-stressed conditions by 2025[9] (see figure 2);

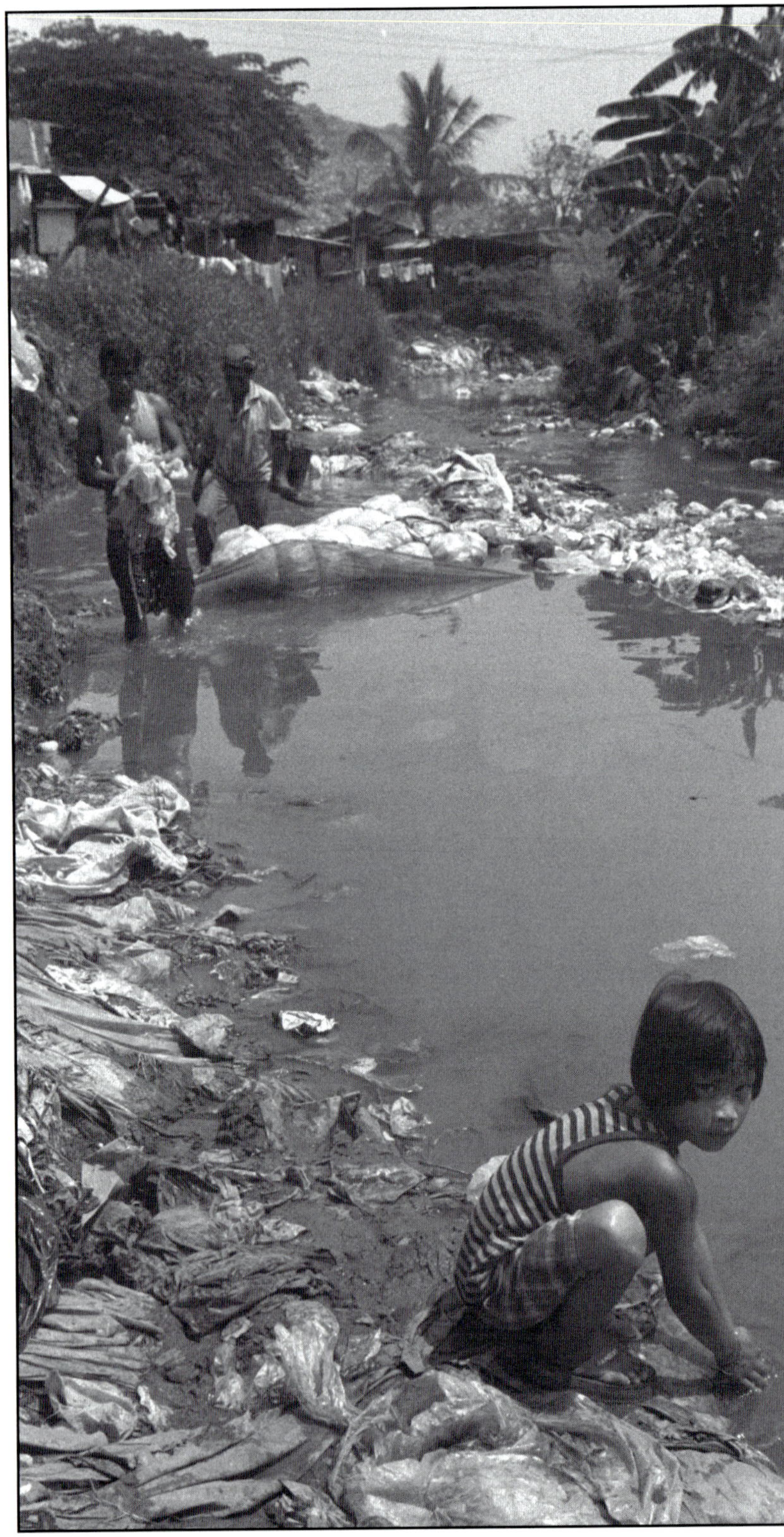

The unsustainable management of chemicals and hazardous wastes is exacting a heavy toll on human health.

- With 70 per cent of the world's drylands degraded, land degradation has negated many advances made by increased agricultural productivity[10];
- Air pollution is at a crisis point in many major cities with over one billion urban residents who breathe unhealthy air[11];
- Climate change is altering weather patterns and disturbing life-supporting natural systems and processes;
- Forests and marine fisheries have been over-exploited; numerous plant and animal species will be lost forever;
- The unsustainable management of chemicals and hazardous wastes is exacting a heavy toll on human health.

Figure 2: Projected global water stress, 2025

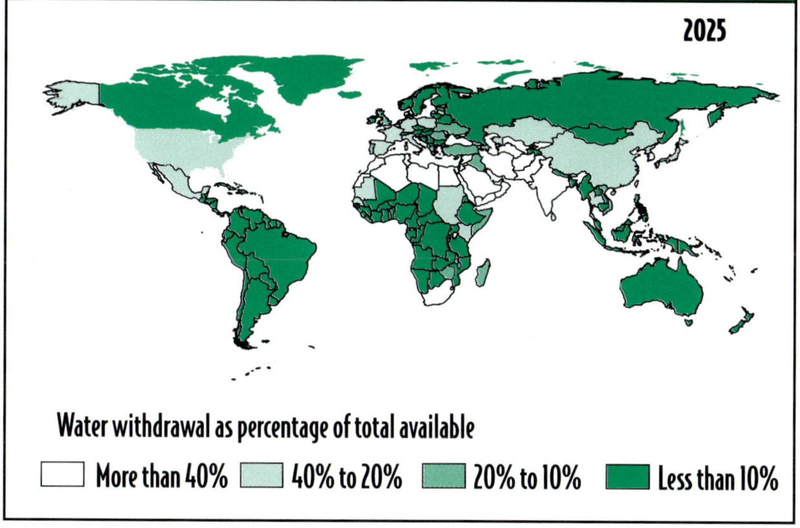

Source: World Meteorological Organization (WMO) and others, Comprehensive Assessment of the Freshwater Resources of the World, WMO, Geneva, 1997.

Note: water stress in the above map is defined as: 'low' when less than 10 per cent of total available is withdrawn; 'moderate' when 10 to 20 per cent of total available is withdrawn; 'medium-high' when 20 to 40 per cent of total available is withdrawn; and 'high' when more than 40 per cent of total available is withdrawn.

Such environmental degradation continues to be a powerful contributor to many current pressing global health threats. Tragically, it is often children who succumb to environmental health threats. For example, acute respiratory infections (ARI), often caused by bacteria that thrive in unclean environments, are the biggest cause of childhood mortality. The highest incidence of ARI is in developing countries[12]. Furthermore, diarrhoeal diseases claim nearly two million children under five every year and malaria continues to debilitate and kill in many countries[13].

The linkages between environmental degradation and health will be one of the issues discussed at the World Summit on Sustainable Development, to be held in Johannesburg, South Africa in August 2002. The Summit will review how the commitments made at UNCED have been implemented. It will also provide an important opportunity for the international community to inject a new spirit of cooperation and urgency based on agreed actions in the common quest for sustainable development.

Environmental Risks to Children's Health

Environmental conditions that are harmful to human health are termed "environmental threats" or "environmental risks" and include such factors as air quality, water quality and specific pollutants. Health threats due to behavioural and lifestyle patterns, such as smoking, unbalanced diets, lack of exercise and drug use could also be considered as "environmentally" related, but fall beyond the scope of this book.

Environmental threats to human health can broadly be divided into "traditional" hazards, stemming largely from a lack of development, and "modern" hazards, arising essentially from unsustainable patterns of development.

Traditional environmental health hazards remain the primary source of ill-health today for the majority of world population: biologically contaminated water, poor sanitation, indoor smoke, rampant disease vectors such as mosquitoes, deficient food hygiene and unsafe waste disposal are usually associated with poverty and social exclusion.

Modern environmental health hazards are closely associated with unsustainable patterns of production and consumption. Typical "modern" environmental problems include, air, water and soil pollution, unsafe use of chemicals, inadequate solid and hazardous waste management, climate change, ozone layer depletion and acid rain due to the use of fossil fuels. In rapidly industrializing countries, modern hazards often compound the traditional health threats.

The quality of the environment and the care a child receives from parents and family members exerts a powerful influence on whether a child survives his or her first years and subsequently influences his or her physical and mental development processes. Figure 3 shows the top killers of children, with acute respiratory infections, diarrhoeal diseases and malaria accounting for approximately 40 per cent of under-five child death. These three categories of disease are closely related to environmental factors, as shown in the first data column in table 1. Overall, environmental conditions are responsible for 33 per cent of the global burden of disease. As illustrated in table 1, 15.4 per cent of the global burden of disease associated with environmental factors is borne by children under the age of 15. This child component of environmental global burden of disease, measured by the loss of disability-adjusted life years (DALYs), represents about two-thirds of the total environment-related DALYs. Taking action to reduce environmental threats could make a major contribution to child health.

The quality of the environment and the care a child receives from parents and family members exerts a powerful influence on whether a child survives his or her first years.

Figure 3: Top killers of children

Under-five deaths by cause, 1999

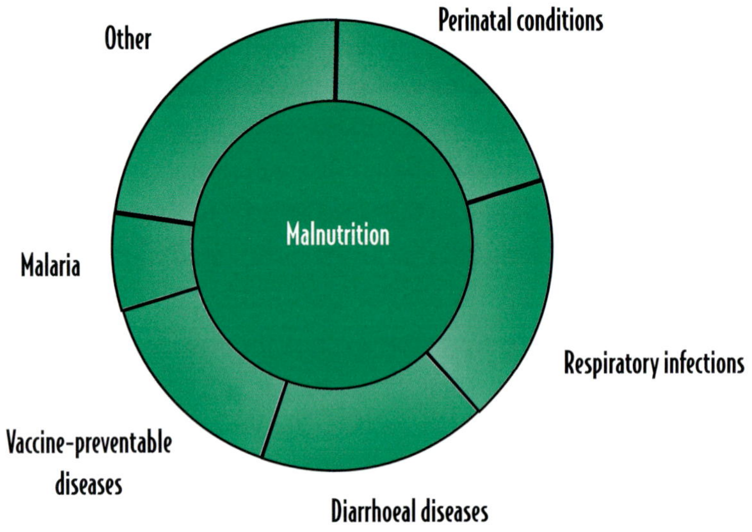

Source: United Nations Children's Fund (UNICEF), Progress since the World Summit for Children: A Statistical Review, page 3, UNICEF, New York, September 2001.

Note: Although the total of under-five deaths is relatively well known, the proportion related to each cause is much more uncertain and hence no numbers are used on the chart. Malnutrition is associated with half of all deaths.

1.2 billion people still struggle to survive with less than $1 a day, at least half of them children.

Underlying Causes of Children's Environmental Health Problems

Poverty remains a primary root cause

Poverty, widespread in the developing world, is an underlying cause of both the ill-health and under-nourishment of children. It also contributes to the deterioration of natural resources and the environment. In industrialized countries, poverty is found in pockets, typically in urban centres, with similar consequences as in developing countries. Today, with a $30 trillion global economy, 1.2 billion people still struggle to survive on less than $1 a day, at least half of them children[14]. Even in the world's richest countries, one in every six children lives below the national poverty line[15].

In ecologically fragile areas, for instance in arid or near-desert areas, or in flood-prone places, low-lying regions, remote mountainous terrain, overcrowded urban slums, or refugee camps, natural resources are scarce and environmental conditions arduous. In these places-- mostly inhabited by poor people -- the toll of environment-related diseases is highest.

Poverty exposes children to terrible risks to their health and development.

Poverty robs children of the right to grow to their full potential. Childhood is a time of rapid growth and development, when great leaps are made physically, intellectually and emotionally. It is also a time of great vulnerability to environmental risks that can lead to illness, permanent physical and mental problems or death. Poverty exposes children to terrible risks to their health and development.

The gap between the richest and the poorest of the world has continued to widen and inequality across nations has steadily increased since 1980[16]. Serious disparities also exist within countries. Both globally and within most countries, a small proportion of the population consumes a much larger share of natural resources than their poor counterparts. Over-consumption, both in terms of the level and pattern, intensifies poverty and aggravates environmental pollution. To reduce poverty requires not only economic growth, according to research, but also disparity reduction measures, such as explicit policy and strong leadership on children's issues, good governance, proper economic incentives, sufficient investment in basic social services and sound environmental management. Developing countries around the world face the challenge of speeding economic growth while slowing environmental degradation. They, therefore, need help in coordinating and integrating economic and environmental policies to achieve sustainable development.

Table 1. Global Burden of Diseases (DALYs)[a] associated with environmental exposures in children under Age 15 – 1990

Diseases	Environmental fraction of global burden of disease (%)[b]	Child portion (C) and total (T) environmental DALYs (1,000 years)[c]	% of all DALYs[d]	
			All age groups	Age 0-14 years
Diarrhoeal diseases	90	84,100 (C) 89,670 (T)	6.5	6.1
Malaria	90	24,400 (C) 28,535 (T)	2.1	1.8
Acute respiratory infections	60	63,000 (C) 70,017 (T)	5	4.6
Chronic respiratory diseases	50	7,700 (C) 30,185 (T)	2.2	0.56
Unintentional injuries	30	22,400 (C) 45,656 (T)	3.3	1.6
Cancer	25	1,500 (C) 17,628 (T)	1.3	0.11
Vaccine-preventable infections	10	6,900 (C) 7,117 (T)	0.5	0.5
Tuberculosis	10	530 (C) 3,843 (T)	0.3	0.04
Mental health	10	1,100 (C) 14,495 (T)	1.1	0.08
Cardiovascular diseases	10	1,600 (C) 13,324 (T)	1	0.12
Overall[e]	33	213,230 (C) 320,470 (T)	23	15.5

Sources: World Health Organization (WHO), Health and Environment in Sustainable Development: Five Years after the Earth Summit, tables 5.3 and 5.14, WHO, Geneva, 1997. Murray CJL and Lopez AD, The Global Burden of Disease, Harvard School of Public Health, WHO, World Bank, 1996. (Figures under revision)

a. Global burden of disease is measured by DALYs, disability-adjusted life years. Each DALY indicates the loss of a year of healthy life – that is, time lived with a disability or time lost through premature death.
b. The percentages reflect how important environmental factors are in causing the burden of a disease and indicate how much their control would contribute to its reduction.
c. Global burden of disease in children associated with environmental exposures in this disease category, measured by DALY.
d. The burden of each disease associated with environmental exposures, as a percentage of the global burden of all diseases.
e. Percentage numbers in this row are not the sum of respective column.

In spite of the many new opportunities globalization brings, it has tended to deepen economic disparity within and between nations.

The influence of global trends

Among the trends influencing the phenomenon of poverty in today's world, globalization and urbanization are perhaps the most significant ones, with the latter having a particularly direct impact on children.

In spite of the many new opportunities globalization brings, it has tended to deepen economic disparity within and between nations. As the Secretary-General of the United Nations Kofi Annan has pointed out, "Millions are experiencing globalization not as an opportunity, but as a force of disruption or destruction: as an assault on their material standards of living, or on their traditional way of life."[17] The scale of the impact that globalization will create on the world's environment and children's well-being, and the exact forms such impact will take, are yet to be seen and further evaluated.

In the course of the last century, urbanization has led to the concentration of half of humanity in cities around the world. In most developing countries, this means the populations of their main cities far outstrip the capacities of urban infrastructures and basic services (see box 3). One quarter to one third of all urban households in the world live in absolute poverty[18], according to estimates. In Africa, cities have the highest rate of poverty of all regions: 40 per cent and rising[19].

Degraded environmental conditions and other physical hazards are common and inescapable for the poor in densely populated cities.

Degraded environmental conditions and other physical hazards are common and inescapable for the poor in densely populated cities, where infectious disease can spread rapidly. It is estimated that at least 220 million people in the cities of the developing world lack access to clean drinking water, 420 million have no access to even simple latrines, and over a billion urban residents are exposed to health-threatening levels of pollution[20]. Additionally, pollution from traffic and industries is prevalent to urban settings. Large numbers of adolescents face particular threats with little or no support (see figure 4).

Figure 4: Moving to the cities

Adolescent populations in developing countries by urban and rural areas, 1990-2025

[population aged 10to19, in millions]

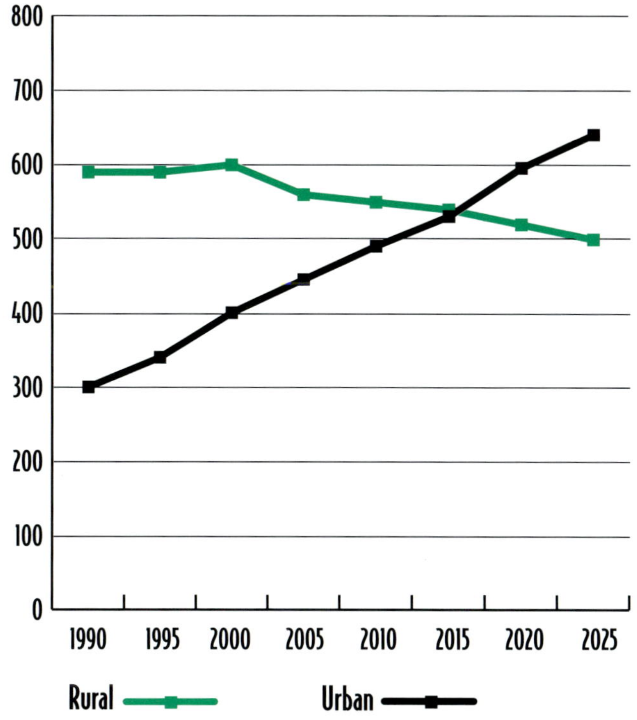

The largest generation in history will soon be the most urbanized. Moving to the city may mean:

- Growing exposure to risks, such as alcohol and drugs, violence and HIV/AIDS
- Loss of culture and isolation from extended family
- Improved access to better schools
- More employment opportunities
- Falling birth rates (over time)

Source: United Nations Children's Fund (UNICEF), The Progress of Nations 1998, New York, UNICEF, 1998.

Box 3: Life in the Slums

The lack of affordable housing for low-income urban households in developing countries has resulted in a proliferation of slums and squatter settlements. There are many characteristics common to life in urban poverty: an appalling reality for one-fourth to one-third of all urban households in the world.

Roots: Most urban slum and shantytown dwellers were originally from rural areas and were driven to towns and cities by poverty.

Youth: Because rural migrants to cities and towns continue to have the large families common in the countryside, the average age of slum inhabitants is very low.

Overcrowding and Squalor: Population density in slums is the highest in the world. Overcrowding, lack of safe water, and inadequate waste disposal, drainage and sanitary systems create conditions hazardous to health.

Women householders: Women-headed households are among the poorest and typically represent a high proportion of those in informal settlements worldwide.

No services: Most slum households must fetch their water from a standpipe and deposit their waste in open drains.

Malnutrition and disease: Slum dwellers are dependent on cash to secure food. Because incomes are very low, children are malnourished.

Premature adulthood: Children are often pulled out of school to earn extra income. Many are abandoned or leave home.

Polluted environment: Poor cities have some of the worst levels of air pollution in the world.

Sources: Compilation based on material from the UN Centre for Human Settlements (Habitat), Cities in a Globalizing World – Global Report on Human Settlements 2001; Earthscan Publications, London, 2001; and UNCHS; the State of the World's Cities 2001, UNCHS, Nairobi 2001.

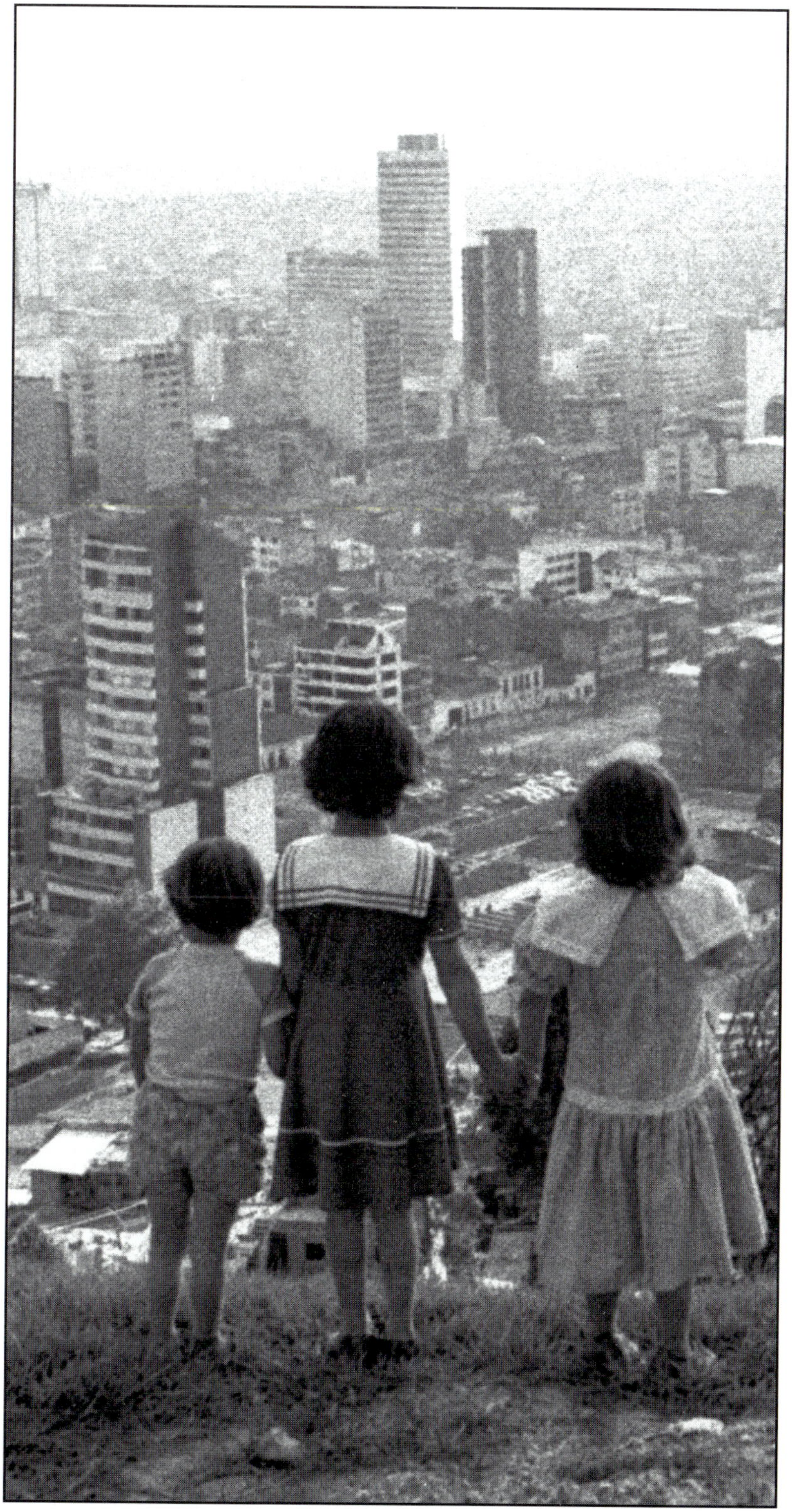

In the course of the last century, urbanization has led to the concentration of half of humanity in cities around the world.

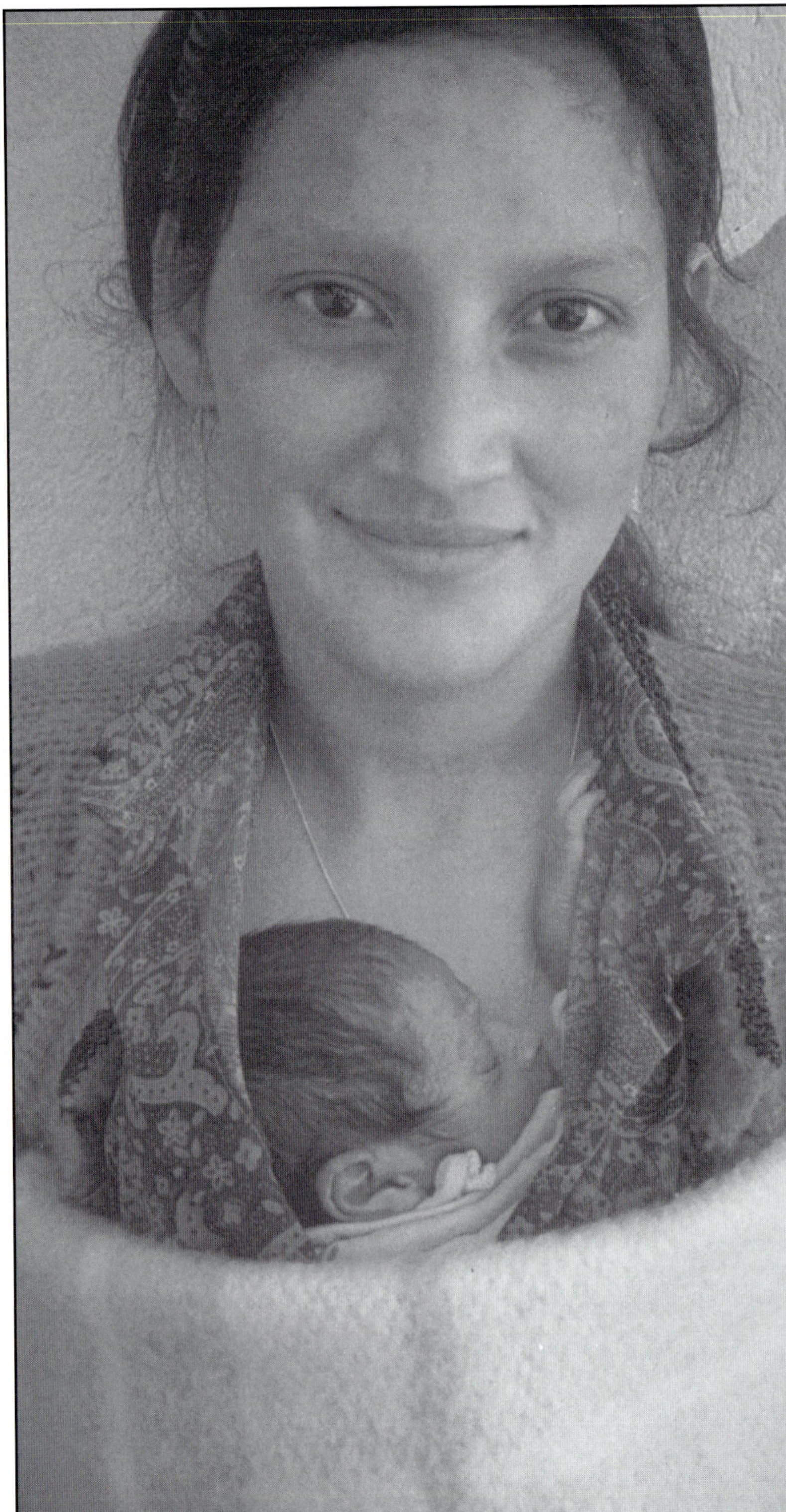

The environment influences children at all stages of their lives, before birth and in their homes, schools and communities.

2 A Child's World and Life Cycle

Children require the care, love and stimulation of parents and families, as well as the best and safest of environments to survive and develop to their full potential.

The environment influences children at all stages of their lives, before birth and in their homes, schools and communities. They are affected by media such as water, air, food, objects or soil; and they are affected by their daily activities or circumstances, including eating, drinking, working and playing (see figure 5).

As children develop and grow, they interact with and explore a world that can offer either an array of life-enhancing discoveries and opportunities or a series of perils that can cause disease and suffering.

This chapter reviews children's special vulnerability and susceptibility to environmental threats at their each developmental stage. A more detailed discussion of key environmental hazards is presented in Chapter 3.

Pregnancy

A woman's health directly influences the health and development of her child. Ensuring that pregnancies are healthy can be of profound benefit to women, children and society at large. It is now recognized that perinatal conditions, many of which are significantly influenced by environmental conditions, account for 20 per cent of the under-five mortality rate worldwide[1]. It is also recognized that a woman's well-being helps determine the well being of

Figure 5: How Children Are Exposed to Environmental Risks

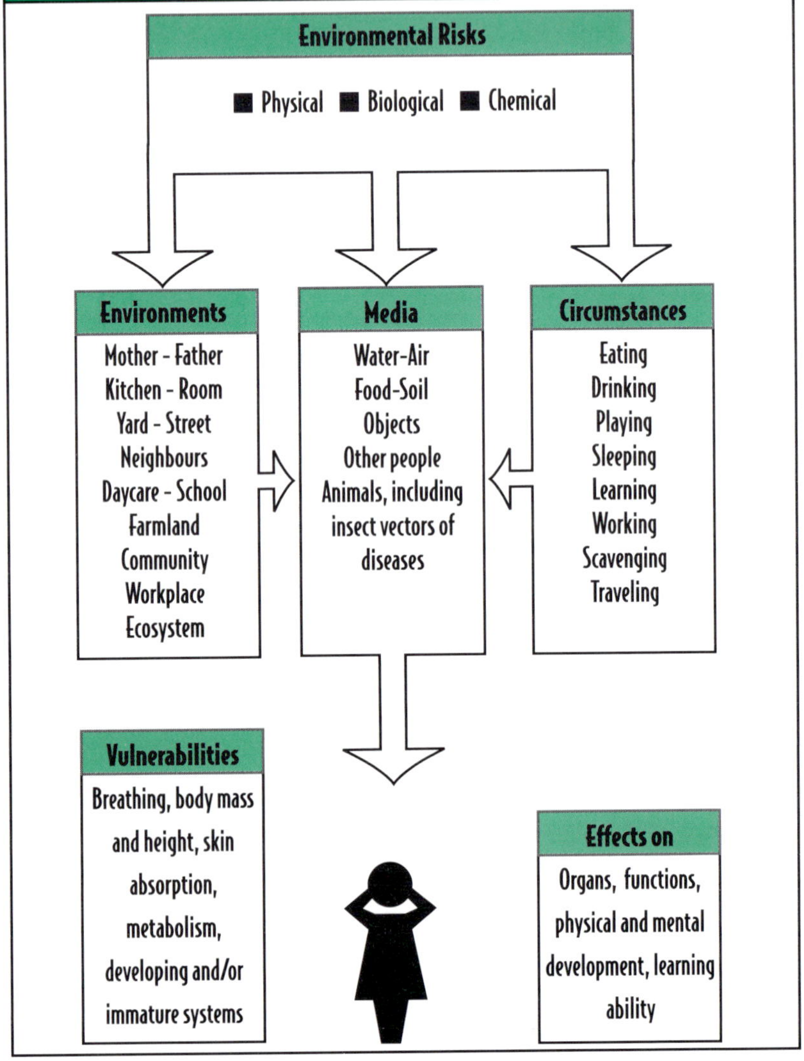

Source: adapted from the World Health Organization

her entire family. A healthy mother is better able in all ways to care for her family and participate fully in the life of her society.

Protein energy malnutrition in pregnant women is a significant threat, causing anaemia, which can severely impact a foetus' growth and development. An expectant mother's malnourishment can result in long-term consequences for her child's development. It has been estimated that eliminating malnutrition among pregnant women would reduce disabilities among their infants by almost one third[2].

Another risk comes from the presence of parasitic worms in the pregnant woman, which can adversely affect or even kill the developing foetus. Approximately 44 million pregnant women in developing countries have hookworm infections[3], which are directly related to environmental factors such as waste disposal.

An expectant mother's malnourishment can result in long-term consequences for her child's development.

Congenital abnormalities are the second leading cause of death in high-income countries[4]. In the United States, these anomalies, along with sudden infant death syndrome and premature birth, account for more than 50 per cent of all infant mortalities[5]. Approximately 3 to 10 per cent of these cases have been attributed to exogenous and environmental agents[6].

Women can be exposed to harmful chemicals at home or through their work, and pass them to a foetus, such as in the case of lead exposure, raising the risks of abortion, birth defects, foetal growth retardation and prenatal death[7] (See Chapter 3). Scientific studies reveal that exposure during the early months of pregnancy can lead to an increased likelihood of mental retardation and development disabilities[8].

Infancy and Early Childhood

The metabolic functions of babies and infants are in a dynamic state of development and their nervous, immune, reproductive and digestive systems are not fully developed. A child's lungs continue to develop long after his or her first breath of air. A child's kidneys, which serve as the principal pathway for elimination of most toxicants from the body, do not reach full functional capacity until the child's first birthday[9]. Any irritants, such as air and water pollutants, encountered during these early stages of growth may permanently impair the development of these vital organs.

Children breathe more air, drink more water, and eat more food than adults do per unit body weight, and this higher rate of intake results in greater exposure to the pathogens and pollutants.

Infants may be exposed to chemical pollutants through their mother's breast milk (See Chapter 3). Yet, despite the risks of exposure to chemicals, breast milk remains the most nutritious and safe source of food for infants worldwide. Thus, the need to protect the environment where pregnant mothers live must be emphasized in order to promote healthy lactation.

Children breathe more air, drink more water and eat more food than adults do per unit body weight, and this higher rate of intake results in greater exposure to pathogens and pollutants. Children drink more than two and a half times as much water as adults do and eat three to four times more per unit of body weight than the average adult[10]. Therefore, if the water contains residues of pesticides or other chemicals, infants will receive more than double the dose of an adult drinking the same water[11]. If the level of exposure to pollution continues from infancy onward, they will be at a greater corresponding lifetime risk.

Children in developing countries are some 13 times more likely to die before they reach their fifth birthday than their counterparts in developed countries. There are many biological environmental factors associated with this high toll, among them the lack of clean water and sanitation, as well as environmental-related diseases such as malaria, dengue fever and Japanese encephalitis. (See Chapter 3.)

Children are curious and learn by exploring their world. They are, therefore, in close contact with their environment. Infants, for instance, explore their world by putting their hands and objects in their mouths and are at risk from pathogens and pollutants on these surfaces. Also, because children are small, they are close to the ground, where they also crawl and play and where they can be exposed to dust and chemical particulates that accumulate on floors and soil[12]. Close parental care and supervision is, therefore, crucial to the safe and healthy development of young children.

Medical and educational research has shown that the development of intelligence, personality and social behaviour occurs most rapidly in humans during their first three to four years. It is estimated that half of all intellectual development potential is established by age four[13]. According to recent research, brain development is much more vulnerable to environmental influence than was previously suspected, and the influence of early environmental quality on brain development is long lasting[14].

Psychosocial and cognitive development begins at birth and parents are the children's earliest teachers. Therefore, strengthening the ability of the mother and all family members to care for and stimulate their children and encourage them to learn, can set the stage for adult success[15]. However, the ability to care for children is greatly influenced by the physical environment. In many countries, particularly those where the environment is seriously degraded, collecting water, gathering firewood and tending crops take up large amounts of time and energy. When those tasks fall without relief on women, they have too little time to spend on ensuring the best possible care for their children. When parents are absent or ill, they are unable to keep children safe as they explore their world.

The ability to care for children is greatly influenced by the physical environment.

Children of School Age

More than 1.4 billion children from age five to 14 – approximately 87 per cent of all children – live in developing countries, where many of the biggest environmental challenges exist (see table 2).

School age children's environments expand beyond their homes and care centres, giving them frequent interaction with a wider range of people in more places than when they were younger.

Several potential environmental risks are particularly associated with children in this age period. Helminth diseases, which are caused by intestinal worms found in soils and vegetables, are one of the common health problems among school age children in developing countries. Those children commonly carry up to 1,000 hookworms, roundworms and whipworms at a time, which can cause anaemia and other debilitating conditions[16]. These illnesses can result in impaired learning, poor school performance and more absences from school (see Chapter 3).

Box 4: Environmental Sanitation in Schools

How sanitary can conditions be when 90 young children in a school are sharing one toilet? Or when more than half of the toilets are not functioning? According to a 1995 pilot survey of 14 countries in the developing world, the average number of children to each toilet in the urban schools is often more than 50. None of the 14 countries had increased the number of school toilets by more than 8 per cent since 1990, suggesting that they are barely managing to keep up with the rise in student populations. Inadequate sanitation and water in schools jeopardize not only students' health but also their attendance. Girls in particular are likely to be kept out of school if there are no sanitation facilities.

ource: United Nations Children's Fund, The Progress of Nations 1997. UNICEF, New York, 1997.

Injuries (usually road traffic injuries, falls and drowning) are now the number-one killer of children aged five to 14 years in developed countries[17]. In developing countries, environmental factors such as exposed cooking set-ups, dangerous tools and equipment, open sewers, heavy traffic, dangerous construction or electrical sites and hazardous chemicals pose threats. A child's health and growth may also be affected when he or she engages in wage-earning work or domestic chores unsuitable for his or her age and ability, such as working long hours in a field, carrying heavy loads, and walking long distances for fuel wood or water.

Asthma and childhood cancers are now major concerns in developed countries (see box 10 for asthma). In the United States, cancer is the second biggest killer of children after accidents, with the median age of child victims of cancer being six years old[18]. Acute leukaemia is the most common type of cancer found in children, and its incidence appears to be rising in some developed countries.

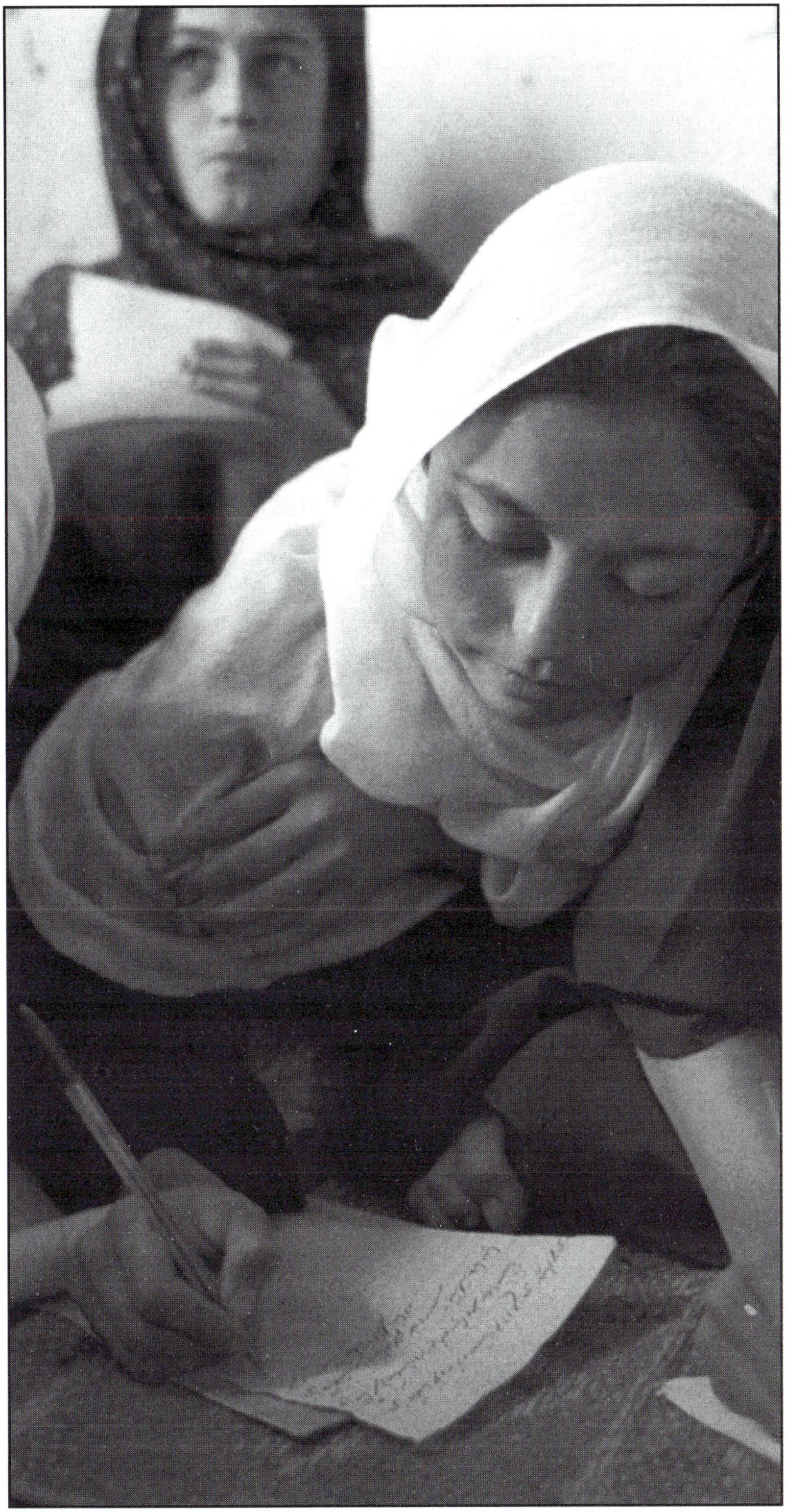

Healthful school environments can raise children's learning opportunities significantly.

Table 2: Leading causes of death, both sexes, 1998 (global)

Rank	0-4 years	5-14 years	15-44 years	45-59 years
1	Perinatal conditions	Acute lower respiratory infections	HIV/AIDS	Ischaemic heart disease
2	Acute lower respiratory infections	Malaria	Road traffic injuries	Cerebrovascular diseases
3	Diarrhoeal diseases	Road traffic injuries	Interpersonal violence	Tuberculosis
4	Measles	Drowning	Self-inflicted injuries	Trachea/ bronchus / lung cancers
5	Malaria	Diarrhoeal diseases	Tuberculosis	Cirrhosis of the liver
6	Congentital abnormalities	War injuries	War injuries	HIV/AIDS
7	HIV/AIDS	Nephritis/ Nephrosis	Ischaemic heart disease	Liver cancers

Source: WHO, World Health Report 1999 Database.
For more data, visit http://www.who.int/whr/1999/en/disease.htm

While the causes remain unclear[19], certain toxic substances and radiation in the environment are believed to be factors in the cell changes that lead to cancer[20]. Among the environmental factors that may play a role are tobacco smoke, radon, asbestos, ultraviolet light radiation, hazardous waste and some pesticides[21].

While not all children are able to attend or remain in school, classrooms are important places for bringing about behavioural changes, promoting better health for students, and teaching about caring for the community environment. Schools have a special role in encouraging urban children to develop a relationship with the natural world. Healthful school environments can raise children's learning opportunities significantly, but often sanitary and environmental conditions in rural and urban schools can be appalling in poor areas, greatly affecting a child's health and learning (see box 4).

Adolescence

During the critical phase of adolescence, the ability of young people to develop their capacities and life skills and to participate meaningfully in society hinges on a number of cultural, socio-economic and environmental factors.

Unsafe schools pose risks for the health and development of many adolescents. Some conditions, such as the lack of proper sanitary facilities or latrines for girls, discourage young women from attending school.

In addition, adolescence is a time when young people often need to work to support their families. Poverty and resource degradation in an adolescent's community can significantly diminish employment possibilities. Hazardous working conditions are also of prime concern for this age group. Adolescents' lighter body weight and lack of skills may predispose them to injuries in the workplace.

One of the gravest risks facing adolescents is that of HIV/AIDS, a major killer in this age group, particularly in sub-Saharan Africa and Asia (see Box 5). HIV/AIDS victims reportedly suffer most from diarrhoeal diseases, to which they succumb more readily due to the weakened state of their immune systems. An improved environment is necessary to protect infected people from other preventable diseases that are caused by unhygienic and degraded environments and further strain health conditions for people infected with HIV/AIDS.

Children in Need of Special Protection

Every day, children of all ages are exposed to a harsh world, with few or no protections from environmental hazards, ill health and injuries. They may be orphans, or living on the streets, begging or selling goods or even their bodies to survive. Many others labour (see box 6). There are also millions of children and adults with physical and mental disabilities who lack access to basic health, education and other social services, a denial of their rights that increases their vulnerability to environmental risks and hazards.

Approximately half of the worldwide refugee and internally displaced populations are children.

Approximately half of the worldwide refugee and internally displaced populations are children[22]. At least 10 million people are estimated to be environmental refugees, more than half of them believed to be in sub-Saharan Africa[23]. These are people displaced from their homes because of weather-related catastrophes, such as earthquakes, floods and cyclones, degraded land, lack of natural resources to support livelihoods or armed conflict and land mines. In the past decade 2 million children have been killed in armed conflict[24]. Children are hardest hit by all these catastrophes, the ensuing outbreaks of diseases and famines in refugee conditions, and the associated psychological traumas.

Box 5: HIV/AIDS and Adolescents

In sub-Saharan Africa and Asia, the impact of HIV/AIDS on adolescents threatens to devastate entire communities, rolling back decades of development and progress. There are 11.8 million young people (15-24 of age) living with HIV/AIDS as of end 2001, of which 8.6 million in sub-Saharan Africa and 1.84 million in Asia. Among those HIV/AIDS affected young people, 7.3 million were women and 4.5 million men, indicating a greater risk faced by young women.

Furthermore,

- 500,000 children died of AIDS in 2000, bringing the total to 4.3 million who have died since the beginning of the pandemic.
- AIDS has orphaned at least 10.4 million children currently under 15 (that is, they have lost their mother or both parents to the epidemic).
- Half of all new infections – almost 6,000 daily – are occurring among young people under the age of 25.
- 2.5 million children at risk of HIV infection through mother-to-child transmission.
- Surveys in 20 developing countries reveal that over half of adolescents have never heard about AIDS or do not know that HIV cannot be transmitted through mosquitoes.

Sources: United Nations Children's Fund and Joint United Nations Programme on HIV/AIDS (UNAIDS), No Time to be Young in a World with AIDS, Poster, UNICEF and UNAIDS, New York, 2001; and UNAIDS and World Health Organization, AIDS Epidemic Update, WHO, Geneva, 2000.

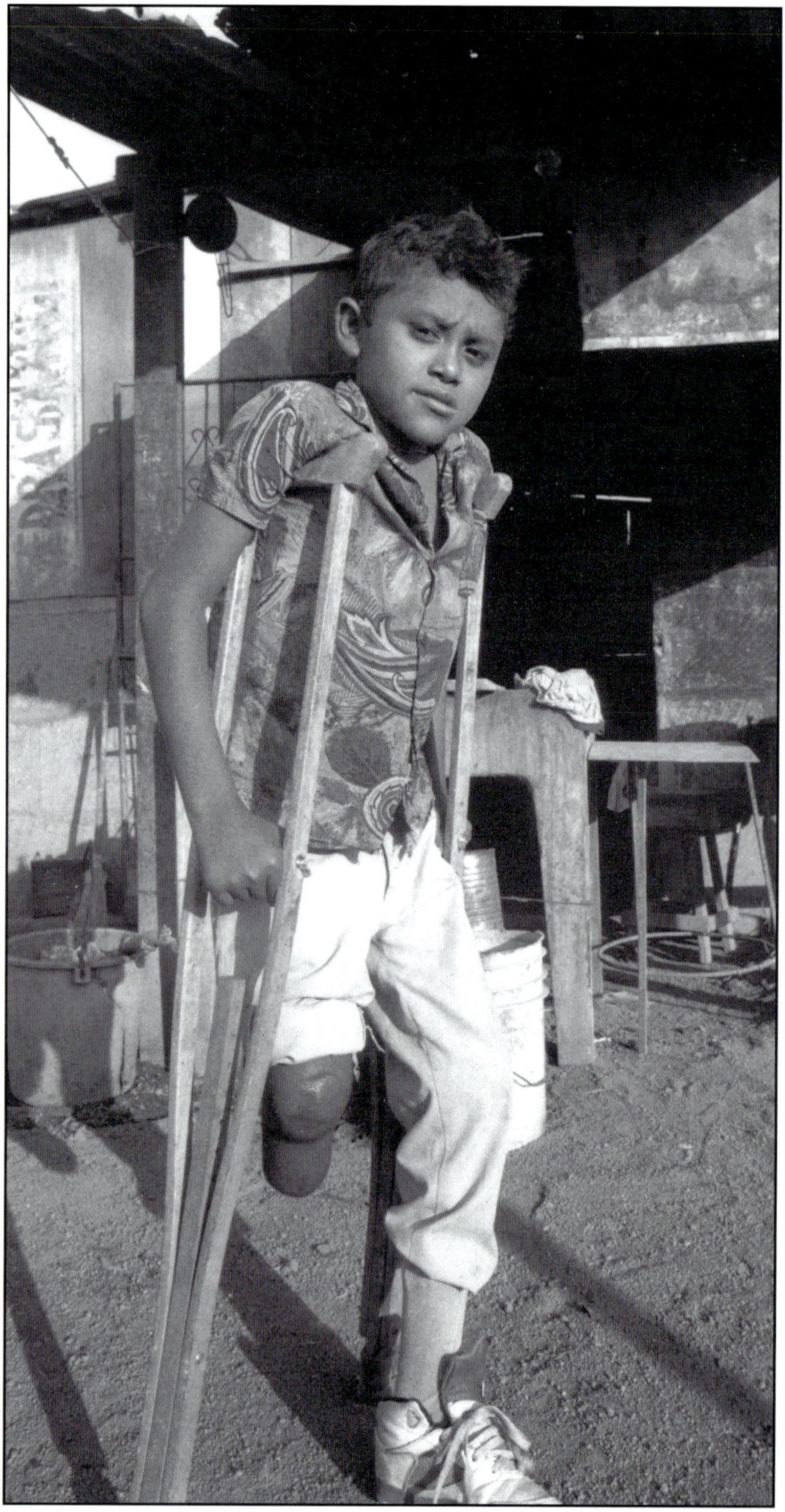

In the past decade two million children have been killed in armed conflict.

Box 6: Child Labour

Extreme poverty often forces children to work to help their families to survive. Work places that use child labour are often congested, dusty, inadequately ventilated and, in some instances, require the handling of chemicals.

It has been estimated that during 1997-98, some 250 million children five to 14 years old were toiling in economic activities in developing countries and almost 70 per cent of them work in dangerous environments with threats to their health, safety and cultural values. For close to half of them, this work was carried out on a full-time basis, while for the remaining half it was combined with schooling or other non-economic activities. As much as 69 per cent of working children were affected by various hazards, and from five per cent to more than 20 per cent of whom suffered actual injuries, with some forced to stop working permanently.

The primary illnesses and injuries were punctures, broken or complete loss of body parts, burns and skin disease, eye and hearing impairment, respiratory and gastro-intestinal illnesses, fever and headaches from excessive heat in the fields or in factories.

Half of working children laboured for nine hours or more a day, with up to four-fifths of these children working seven days a week. The child worker has a high risk of burns, falls, chemical poisoning, lung diseases, etc. Also, because their bodies are not fully developed and their young minds perhaps unaware of the dangers, they are more likely to be injured or to become ill.

The 1999/2000 Multiple Indicator Cluster Surveys (MICS) of 49 developing countries revealed that 23 per cent of rural children (5-14 years old) worked, as compared to 13 per cent in urban areas. Saharan African countries showed the highest proportion of children working.

Sources: Statistics on Working Children and Hazardous Child Labour in Brief. International Labour Organisation; and United Nations Children's Fund, UNICEF End Decade Databases – Child work.

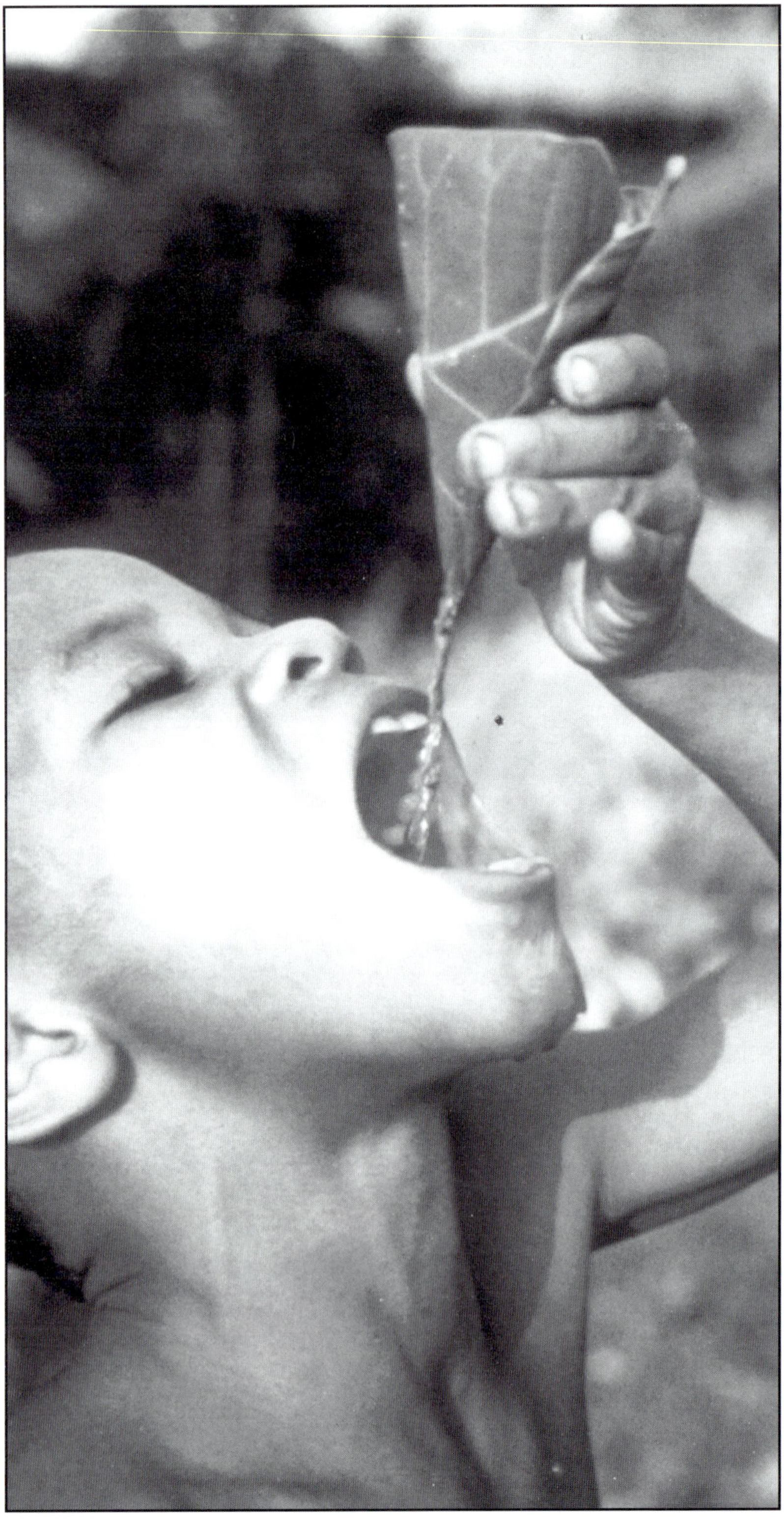

Water is life.

3 Environmental Threats to Children

As discussed above, children are immersed in a world of constant threats to their health and well being. This chapter looks at specific threats of major importance to children, including water and sanitation, chemical pollution, air pollution and natural resource degradation. The next chapter looks at certain global environmental issues, such as climate change and the impact they have on our children's health.

Lack of Safe Water and Sanitation

Water quality and quantity

Water is life. It is essential for sustaining basic human functions, health and food production, as well as for preserving the integrity of the world's ecosystems. Access to safe drinking water is a basic right for all human beings. A child's well-being is highly dependent on both the quality and the availability of water and how well we manage this precious resource.

Around the world, both biological contaminants and chemical pollutants are compromising water quality. This section focuses on biological contaminants, as these cause a series of deadly childhood illnesses in developing countries. Some important chemical pollutants in water will be discussed in the following section.

Biological contaminants of water sources, also called pathogens, include parasites, bacteria and viruses. They get into drinking water when the water source is contaminated by waste material, such as human or animal waste and sewage. The most important source of water contamination in developing countries is human faeces, due to the lack of adequate sanitation facilities. Today, about 2.4 billion people do not have access to even a simple latrine[1]. As a result, human waste heavily pollutes many rivers and lakes in developing countries. For example, in Asia's major rivers, faecal coliform counts can be 50 times higher than the guidelines set by WHO[2]. Children face dangerous health risks when come into contact with such water through washing, bathing or drinking.

Low or non-existent capacity in wastewater treatment is another major factor causing water pollution in most parts of the developing world. In Latin America, only about 14 per cent of urban wastewater receive proper treatment before discharge. Although the level of sewage treatment is reported to be higher among Asian cities (on average about 35 per cent), it is still unacceptable that most of the wastewater is directly drained to various water bodies[3]. Standard wastewater treatment is almost non-existent in many African cities[4].

Moreover, poor water management strategies, combined with habitat modifications (such as land conversion and forest clearance for roads and agriculture), and changing ecological conditions also give rise to water quality degradation and consequent increased vector-borne disease transmissions. The construction of dams and reservoirs, inadequate drainage in irrigation schemes or poor urban water management creates increased quantities of standing surface water. These stagnant water bodies provide the ideal breeding grounds for mosquitoes, which carry various deadly or debilitating diseases, such as malaria.

The amount of water available is as important as its quality.

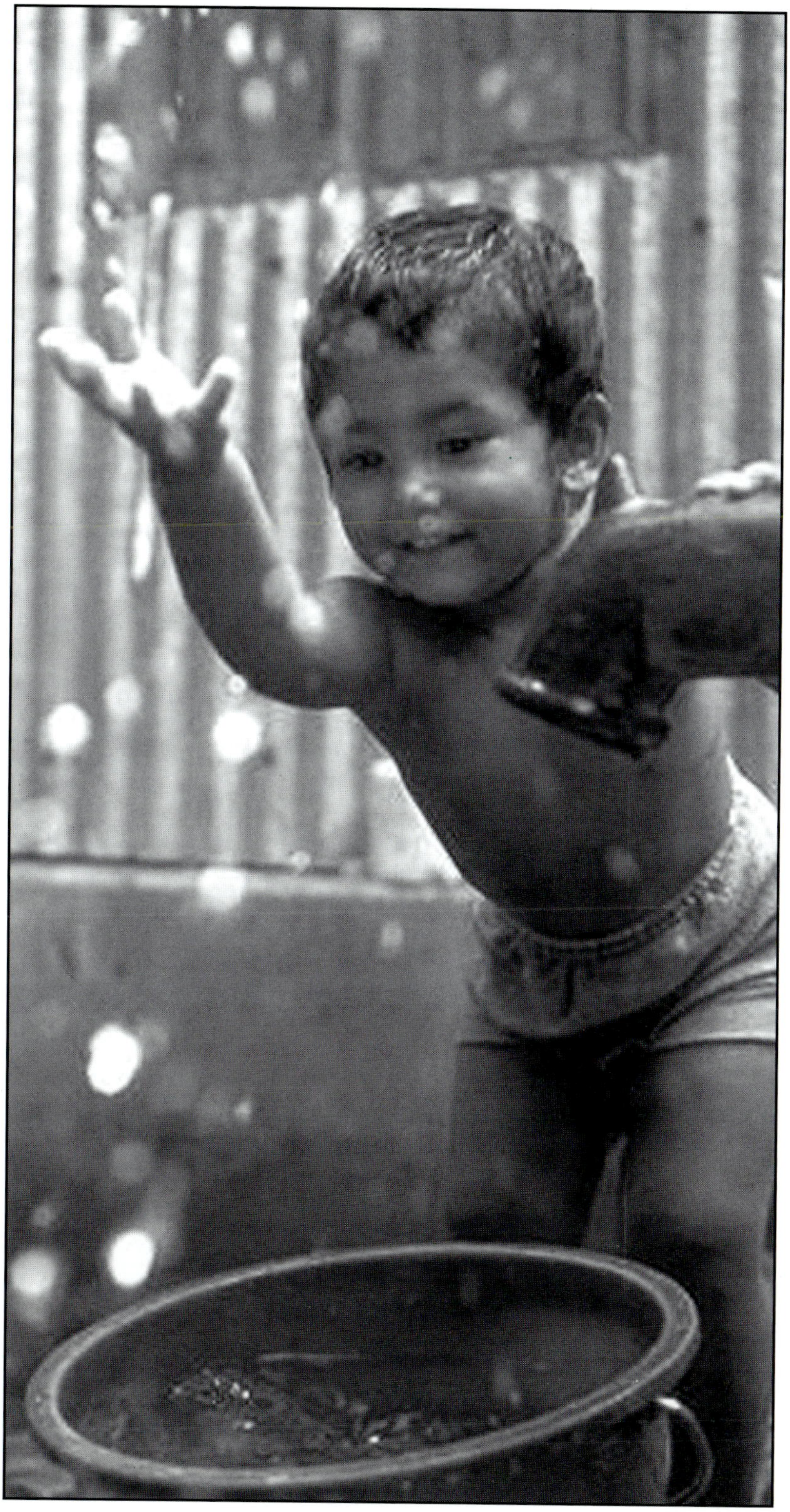

The amount of water available is as important as its quality.

Already, one-third of the world's population lives in countries facing moderate to high water stress and water tables are falling on every continent[5]. If present trends continue, it is estimated that two out of three people on earth will live in water-stressed conditions by 2025[6]. Even where water quantity is not a concern, rural and low-income population's access to safe drinking water poses a major challenge. Globally, 1.1 billion people are without access to clean water supply, such as groundwater drawn from a borehole or protected dug well, rainwater, or protected spring[7]. Too little water makes it virtually impossible to maintain the necessary sanitary conditions in the home, which can lead to the outbreak of debilitating or fatal diseases for children.

Sanitation

Poor sanitation is common in most developing countries. Human excreta, including that of children, contain all sorts of microorganisms from parasite eggs to viruses (see box 7). Unsanitary conditions and practices at the household level, such as absence of sanitary latrines, unsafe waste disposal and unhygienic behaviour in childcare and food preparation, create a dangerous environment with health risks to children. A lack of sanitation facilities in schools helps transmit diseases and keeps millions of girls out of school.

Unsanitary conditions and practices at the household level, create a dangerous environment with health risks to children.

Waste dumps sit in the outskirts of almost all major cities in developing countries, creating not only an unsightly view and unpleasant smells, but also hazardous environmental conditions to those living nearby. While relatively few scientific studies have been conducted regarding adverse health effects of waste landfill sites[8], a recent study found that living near a landfill can raise the risk of having a child with birth defects such as Downs Syndrome by as much as 40 per cent

Selected Facts

- At the dawn of the 21st Century, about 18 per cent of the world's people do not have access to safe drinking water, and nearly 40 per cent lack adequate sanitation[10].
- In Africa, 30 per cent of the rural water supplies are not functioning at any one time. In Asia and Latin America and the Caribbean, the numbers are respectively, 17 per cent and four per cent[11].
- Only about 35 per cent of the urban wastewater was treated in Asia in 2000 and 14 per cent in Latin America. Only a negligible percentage of treatment was reported for Africa[12].
- In large cities of developing countries, the percentage of unaccounted-for water is around 40 per cent, while often below quality standards[13].
- Diarrhoeal diseases claim the lives of nearly 2 million children every year and have killed more children in the last 10 years than all people lost to armed conflict since World War II[14]. In 1998, over 99 per cent of these deaths (for children under 14 years of age) occurred in developing countries[15].
- In 1998, malaria killed more than 1 million children under the age of 15, and was the second leading cause of death in the world for the five-to-14 age group[16]. Sub-Saharan African countries are the worst hit worldwide, where nine out of 10 malaria cases occur[17].
- Schistosomiasis affects over 200 million people worldwide, of whom 88 million are under 15 years of age, with the heaviest infections being reported in the 10-to-14 age group in Africa and South America[18].
- Globally, dengue hemorrhagic fever (DHF) has re-emerged as a major cause of hospitalization and death over the past 20 years. This is partly due to insecticide-resistant vectors and reduced preventive measures, such as environmental controls of vectors. In 1998, more than 2.5 billion people

lived in areas of risk. Each year, there are approximately 50 to 100 million cases of dengue fever and 500,000 cases of DHF[19].

Health impact of unsafe water and poor sanitation

Contaminated water causes a range of diseases which are often life threatening (see box 8). Of the water-borne diseases affecting children, the most deadly are diarrhoeal infections. Children are the most frequent victims of diarrhoeal diseases, with an estimated 80 to 90 per cent of the disease caused by environmental factors[20]. Depending on the severity of the infection, intestinal diseases can result in poor nutrition, anaemia, retarded growth and death. Although diarrhoeal diseases still account for 17 per cent of childhood mortality[21], wide application of oral rehydration therapy and increased access to sanitation and water supply have resulted in a significant decrease in diarrhoeal disease mortality rates for children under five in certain areas of developing countries. Morbidity rates, however, have not decreased largely due to the slow pace of change in hygiene behaviours[22].

Contaminated water causes a range of diseases which are often life threatening.

Cholera, one of the most severe diarrhoeal diseases, is present in faecal-contaminated water. The cholera bacteria thrives best in coastal estuaries and generally only inhabits rivers and other freshwater sources if nutrient levels from organic pollution, such as human faeces, are quite high. Whoever drinks the contaminated water, without treating or boiling it, becomes an ideal candidate for cholera infection and the ensuing fatal dehydration. Children are most susceptible to this disease.

Untreated cholera frequently results in high mortality rates. It is a recurring problem in many areas of the world and has become endemic in some regions. Indeed, the number of reported cases worldwide nearly doubled in 1998 as compared to 1997[23]. In Africa and Latin America, several factors play a role in the dramatic rise in cholera cases: deteriorating water and sanitation systems, poor living conditions, malnutrition or the consumption of contaminated seafood, crowding, use of wastewater to irrigate crops near urban areas, and political and economic turmoil[24].

Box 7: Faeces - the most dangerous pollutant

One gram of human excreta can contain:

- 10,000,000 viruses
- 1,000,000 bacteria
- 1,000 parasite cysts
- 100 parasite eggs

Source: United Nations Children's Fund, Sanitation for All: Promoting Dignity and Human Rights. UNICEF, New York, 2000.

Water-washed diseases arise from insufficient water to permit regular washing of the hands, face, body and clothes, and cause skin and eye infections. For instance, trachoma is an infectious disease associated with dry, arid areas and lack of accessible water supplies. Children are a major reservoir of the trachoma-causing bacteria, but the blindness due to trachoma most frequently occurs in women in their mid-life and beyond. Women have a two to three times higher rate of trachoma and risk of blindness than men, since caring for children is a risk factor for active trachoma and for the progression to trichiasis[25] and blindness[26]. Though the disease-causing bacteria begin in childhood, it progresses over the years as repeated infections cause irritation and scarring on the inside of the eyelid. This infection is easily spread as the children then touch the faces of their mothers and other children. One of the best interventions is surprisingly simple: increase hands and face washing among children.

Water-based diseases are transmitted through aquatic organisms such as aquatic or amphibic snails. The aquatic organisms serve as intermediate hosts to the parasites during certain stages in the life cycle of parasites. In the cases of the schistosome parasite that causes schistosomiasis and the guinea worm the intermediate hosts are small freshwater crustaceans that are ingested in drinking water. Schistosomiasis is detrimental to the growth and develop-

Box 8: Examples of main water-related infections

Waterborne (and water-washed, also food-borne)

- Cholera
- Diarrhoeal diseases
- Enteric fevers: typhoid
- Infective jaundice
- Polio
- Roundworm
- Whipworm

Water-Washed

- Scabies
- Trachoma
- Leishmaniasis
- Typhus
- Lice

Water-Based

- Bilharzia (Schistosomiasis)
- Guinea worm

Water-Related Insect Vector

- Malaria
- Sleeping sickness
- Breakbone fever (Dengue)
- River blindness
- Yellow fever
- Filariasis

Source: Adapted from Satterthwaite, David et al., The Environment for Children. United Nations Children's Fund and Earthscan, New York, 1996.

ment of school-age children and is associated with anaemia, malnutrition and stunting[71]. Guinea worm causes a disfiguring and disabling disease. It breeds in open waters and infects people who drink contaminated water. Fortunately, with decades of concerted effort worldwide, the number of infected people has been drastically reduced, from an estimated 50 million people infected with guinea worm disease in Africa and Asia in the middle of the 20th century to only 96,000 by 1999[28]. This success is attributable to the provision of safe water supplies, identifying and treating of infected people, and effective community monitoring in infested areas. Because of these proactive measures, it is within the realm of possibility that this disease could be completely eradicated in the near future[29].

Several water-related, vector-borne diseases are particularly dangerous to young children, including malaria, Japanese encephalitis and dengue. Malaria occurs in some 100 countries, causing 300 to 500 million acute cases in people each year[30]. In 1998, 90 per cent of deaths were children under 14[31]. In Africa, where 90 per cent of malaria cases occur, the mosquito vector has developed insecticide resistance to one or more insecticides[32] and the parasite's resistance to chloroquine is also widespread. Malarial symptoms include fever and aches, as well as more severe vomiting, diarrhoea, liver and kidney failure, convulsions and death. Children in infected areas can suffer an average of six bouts a year and it is the most common cause of children missing school[33]. In Africa this disease is responsible for an estimated economic loss of $2 billion annually[34].

Several water-related, vector-borne diseases are particularly dangerous to young children.

Japanese encephalitis (JE) endemic regions are mainly in Asia, where high population density puts approximately 3 billion people at risk. Young children under 10 years of age are more likely to die of JE, and if they survive, they are likely to have residual neurological deficits. The disease can have case-fatality rates as high as 30 to 50 per cent. Although a higher case-fatality rate is reported in the elderly, serious neurological and psychiatric permanent effects are more frequent in the very young[35].

The dengue haemorrhagic fever is also a major killer of children, whose mosquito vector has even infested all major urban centres of the American tropics[36].

In developing countries, a lack of water often forces people – usually women and young girls – to spend a lot of time fetching water, often at great distances from the home, or to extract water from alternative, unsafe sources. Lack of access to safe water and sanitation facilities has important implications for the education of children, especially girls since they bear the major burden of carrying the water home from distant sources, preventing them from attending school. In developing countries, lack of sanitation facilities is a major reason for girls dropping out of school. Finally, poor people are more likely required to purchase water at highly elevated costs. When their dwellings are not connected to municipal sources, they are often forced to buy water of doubtful quality from vendors.

In developing countries, lack of sanitation facilities is a major reason for girls dropping out of school.

Taking action

Governments, international organizations, donor agencies and other relevant civil society organizations should strive to:

- Achieve the target set by world leaders at the UN Millennium Summit in September 2000, to halve the percentage of the world's people who are unable to reach or to afford safe drinking water by the year 2015;
- Fulfil the commitment made at the UN Millennium Summit to stop the unsustainable exploitation of water resources, by developing water management strategies at the regional, national and local levels, which promote both equitable access and adequate supplies;
- Strengthen the enforcement of existing environmental regulations on water quality and resource protection; and
- Closely monitor drinking water quality in decentralized supply systems, such as wells and ponds.

Communities should strive to:

- Promote hygiene education and behavioural changes among parents, childcare givers and children, including hand washing as a simple but effective way of blocking hand-to-mouth disease transmissions;
- Develop effective programmes on: school sanitation, proper water handling and storage and protection of water sources.
- Avoid the creation of mosquito breeding grounds through using proper irrigation and drainage techniques, adequate draining in swampy areas, eliminating areas where water

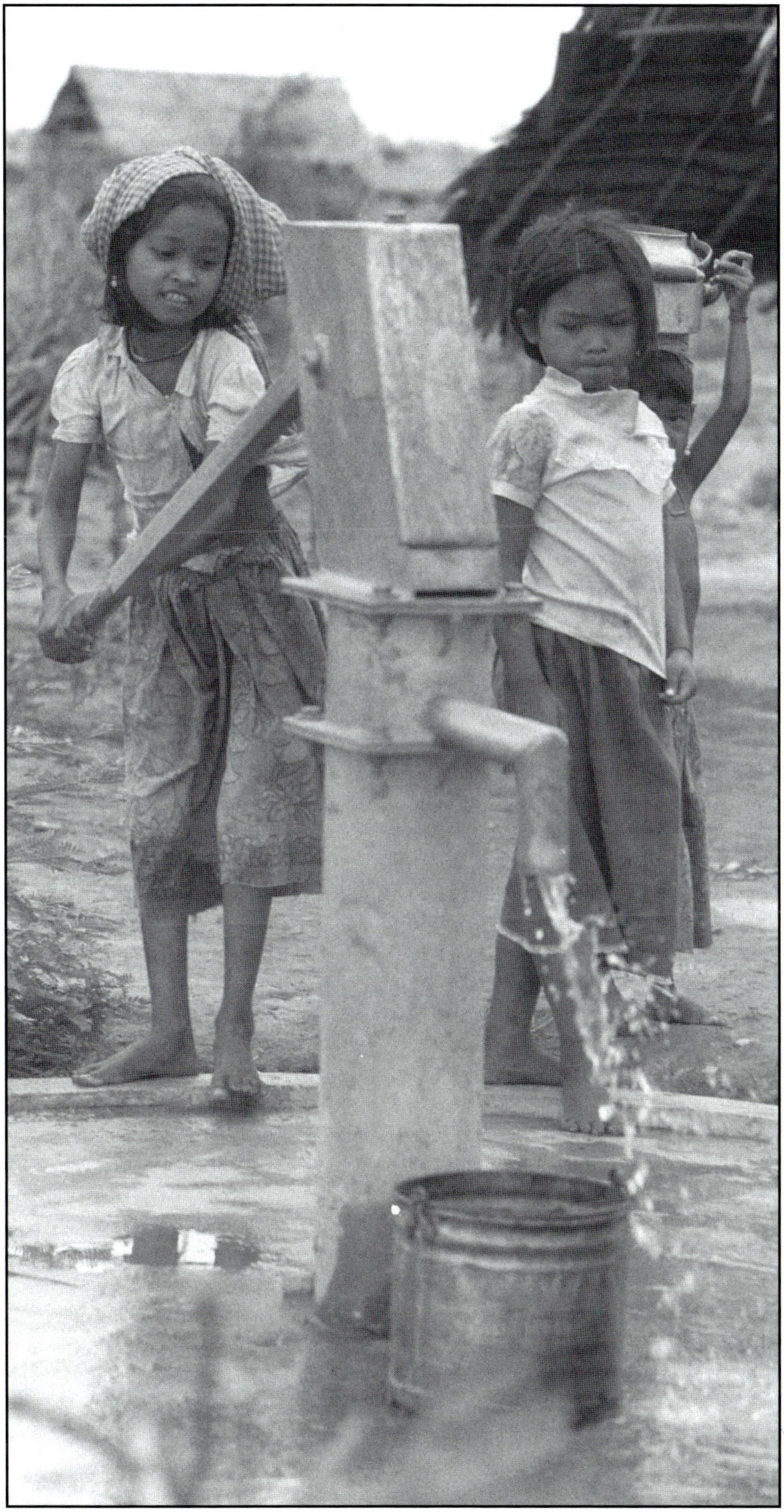

In developing countries, a lack of water often forces people – usually women and young girls – to spend a lot of time fetching water, often at great distances from the home.

collects and stagnates such as discarded tires, improving latrine designs and using sound agricultural practices such as integrated pest management.

Examples of What Works

- The simple act of washing hands with soap and water reduces incidents of diarrhoea from shigella and other causes by up to 35 per cent[37].
- Water, sanitation and hygiene interventions have been shown to reduce sickness from diarrhoea by between 25 per cent and 33 per cent[38].
- Experience shows that communities that have taken health into account have greatly enhanced the efficiency of water projects[39].
- Since children are the most vulnerable to water-related illnesses, their risk factors must be the primary consideration in developing the drinking water standard. As such, the US Environmental Protection Agency's standards for lead, nitrates and nitrites in water are specifically based on risks to children[40].
- Solar water disinfection has proven to be an easy, low-cost, small-scale and immediate technique for providing safe water.
- In Indonesia, when farmers synchronised their rice-production system to allow rice paddies to dry out completely during certain periods, the transmission of malaria was drastically reduced[41].
- In Sri Lanka, the breeding of malaria-transmitting mosquitoes was suppressed in small rivers and irrigation canals by regularly flushing them out[42].

Chemical Pollution and Radiation

The production and use of toxic chemicals pose a major and relatively new threat to humankind and the environment. Synthetic chemicals were virtually unknown at the turn of the last century, but there are now between 50,000 and 100,000 of them being produced commercially. Many of these chemicals have not been thoroughly researched for their effects on human health[43]. Rapid industrialization, urbanization and intensified agriculture all account for the increased chemical pollution worldwide. In certain developing countries, vast amounts of unused pesticides have piled up in storage – some are even stored in houses – and these can pose serious health threats.

Synthetic chemicals were virtually unknown at the turn of the last century, but there are now between 50,000 and 100,000 of them being produced commercially.

The emissions from cars, industrial processes, waste treatment processes, such as incinerators, hazardous materials and the excessive use of pesticides and fertilisers for agricultural and domestic purposes, all release toxic substances into the air, food or water (see tables 3 and 4). Heavy metals and persistent organic pollutants (POPs), such as polychlorinated biphenyls (PCBs), dioxins and DDT, are of particular concern since they do not degrade in the environment for decades and accumulate in, and are toxic to, plants, fish, animals, and humans. These substances also can travel long distances, easily moving from one medium to another in the environment.

The following chemical pollutants are particularly worth mentioning with regard to children's environmental health.

Pesticides

Since synthetic pesticides were first introduced in the early 1960s, their worldwide consumption has grown markedly, with total consumption reaching 2.6 million metric tons of active ingredients in 1995, increasing at about one per cent per year[44]. Developed countries have been the major users of pesticides, consuming about three-quarters of the world total[45].

Pesticides are integral to agriculture and vector-control programmes worldwide, yet children are uniquely susceptible to the health threats that they pose. Once released in the environment, pesticides can pollute rivers, groundwater, air, soil, and food. Human exposure occurs from breathing, drinking, eating, or through skin absorption.

It is crucial to protect mothers from exposure to toxic agents.

A child's exposure to chemicals can occur as early as the prenatal phase, and during infancy through breast-feeding. Organochlorine pesticide residues present in mothers' milk may pose a potential hazard for breast-fed children[46]. A striking example is the presence of chemicals in the breast milk of the Inuit peoples of the Arctic region. Although the region is largely free from polluting industries, some chemicals entered the ecosystem and accumulate at every stage on their way up the food chain: from plants and fish to seals, whales, polar bears and humans. However, breast milk remains the best source of nutrition for infants and is strongly recommended by UNICEF and WHO. Therefore, it is crucial to protect mothers from exposure to toxic agents.

Synthetic chemicals may interfere with natural processes that regulate growth and development. These chemicals are called endocrine disrupters. Examples of endocrine disrupters are PCBs and DDT. Infants are particularly at risk due to the role the endocrine system plays in young children's growth and development. Research on how endocrine disrupters may damage the ability to fend off diseases, learn, integrate socially and reproduce is steadily advancing.

The impact on human health from pesticide exposure depends on a number of factors, including the kind of pesticide involved and its toxicity, the amount or dose of the exposure, the length of exposure, and the way in which the exposure occurs. Specific effects believed to be linked to pesticide exposure are outlined in box 9.

Lead

Although lead is naturally present in the earth's crust, human activities bring it into air, water, food and soil in an amount up to 300 times greater than its natural occurrence[47]. Lead is often found in:

Box 9: Possible Health Effects of Pesticide Exposure

In addition to acute pesticide poisoning that can result in death, a growing body of epidemiological research and studies of laboratory animals suggest the possible link of long-term exposure to certain pesticides and:

- Abnormal growth and development, and failure to acquire normal organ function;
- Endocrine/hormone disruption: certain pesticides in very small doses may mimic or block hormones or trigger inappropriate hormone activity, which can cause, for example, sterility, lowered sperm counts and breast cancer;
- Impaired development of the nervous system that can result in lowered intelligence and behavioural abnormalities;
- Cancers, including leukaemia, sarcoma, lymphoma, Wilm's (malignant tumour of the kidney) and brain cancer in children. Studies have indicated that the risk of developing cancer might be higher if exposure to carcinogens begins in childhood; and
- Compromised immune system, which in children further exacerbates the risk of infectious disease and cancer, thus increasing mortality rates. This is of special concern in developing countries where people can be simultaneously exposed to both pesticides and infectious pathogens when their immune systems are already compromised by other factors, such as malnutrition.

Sources: United Nations Environment Programme, United Nations Children's Fund, World Health Organization, Food and Agricultural Organization, Childhood Pesticide Poisoning: Information for Advocacy and Action (draft), 2000; and Mott, Lawrie et al., Our Children at Risk: The 5 worst environmental threats to their health. Natural Resource Defense Council, New York, 1997.

- Air, as a result of gasoline additives;
- Dust from soil and airborne pollutants, from agricultural practices, or from parents who bring it into the home after having been exposed to it at work;
- Water from lead pipes and faucets, or from fallout from leaded gasoline which leaches into the groundwater;
- Food, particularly green leafy vegetables, growing near polluted areas;
- Drinks in cans which contain lead;
- Paints, which are the primary source of lead in homes;
- Ceramic ware;
- Folk health remedies with high lead content, especially in developing countries; and
- Lead smelters, incinerators and battery recycling plants.

Lead is a significant child health hazard.

Lead is a significant child health hazard. It can even be a threat before birth. If a pregnant woman is exposed to lead, it can be transferred to the unborn child and cause premature birth, low birth weight, or even abortion. Lead is toxic when ingested and inhaled. Encountered in the environment, it enters the bloodstream, where it reaches the kidneys and the brain and deposits in bones and teeth. Growing epidemiological evidence suggests that lead in a child's body, even in small amounts, can cause disturbances in early physical and mental growth and later in intellectual functioning and academic achievements, hindering the child's ability to reach full potential. Studies have concluded that there is a direct effect of low-level lead exposure on IQ of children. Furthermore, undernourished children are more susceptible to the toxicity of lead and more likely to be adversely affected by lead exposure. This may in part reflect the competition between lead and calcium for absorption, so that diets low in calcium allow greater lead absorption. This has significant implications for children in poor urban communities of developing countries where leaded gasoline is still prevalent and under-nourishment remains a key problem. Specific effects of lead are summarised in table 3.

Since the United Nations Commission for Sustainable Development in 1994 called upon Governments and international institutions to take action to phase out leaded gasoline, some progress has been made. Thirty-six countries had already phased out the use of leaded gasoline by 1999 and this will likely rise to 55 countries by 2005[48]. Many of the countries phasing out the use of leaded gasoline are in the developing world. About 78 per cent of all gasoline sold in the world is currently unleaded and this will likely rise to more than 84 per cent by 2005[49].

Mercury

Mercury is a toxic heavy metal normally existing in liquid or gaseous forms and found in water, air or food, most often in freshwater fish or on coated-seeds. Mercury occurs naturally in the

Table 3: What is Known About Lead and Lead Poisoning?

At low levels, lead poisoning in children causes:	At high levels, lead poisoning in children causes:	Effects of lead poisoning on children can be:
■ Reduction in IQ and attention span; ■ Reading & learning disabilities; ■ Hyperactivity & behavioural problems; ■ Impaired growth; ■ Impaired visual & motor functioning; ■ Hearing loss.	■ Anaemia; ■ Brain, liver, kidney, nerve damage; ■ Coma; ■ Convulsions; ■ Death.	■ Long-term and potentially irreversible; ■ Intensified with repeated exposure & accumulation of lead in body.

Source: United Nations Children's Fund and United Nations Environment Programme, Childhood Lead Poisoning: Information for Advocacy and Action, UNICEF and UNEP, New York, 1997.

environment in very small amounts in oceans, rocks and soils, but it also enters the environment in greater amounts through human activities such as coal-fired power generation, waste incineration, certain manufacturing processes, mining activities and medical and dental uses. Mercury is also used in some common household products including fluorescent lights, thermostats, thermometers, and even in some children's toys. At school, mercury may be used in science and chemistry labs, the nurse's office and electrical systems. Methylmercury, an organic mercury compound, is more readily absorbed by humans than elemental mercury and thus is more toxic.

The most common way of exposure to methylmercury is from eating fish from contaminated areas. Methylmercury can be found in freshwater and saltwater fish[50]. In January 2001, the US Environmental Protection Agency (US/EPA) and the US Food and Drug Administration (US/FDA) issued advice to women who are pregnant or may become pregnant, nursing mothers and young children to limit consumption of certain fish to one meal per week because of a concern for mercury contamination. Although fish can be an important source of nutrition for developing children, some fish, such as shark, swordfish, mackerel and tuna, may contain high levels of mercury[51].

Mercury is a potent neurotoxin pollutant, which passes more easily into the brains of the foetus and young child. The developing brain is particularly sensitive to methylmercury. Depending on the dose and exposure level, to varying degrees it can interfere with brain development and cause mental retardation, cerebral palsy and seizures[52]. Mercury may cause cancer and damage the stomach, large intestine and lung. It also may permanently harm unborn children[53].

Nitrates

Nitrate pollution is now considered to be one of the most serious water quality problems in the world[54]. Nitrogen is a basic ingredient in artificial fertilisers. The use of fertilisers has been rapidly increasing, causing excessive nitrogen loading of the environment on a global scale[55]. Global fertiliser use soared from less than 14 million tonnes in 1950 to 135 million tonnes in 1996[56]. As a result, nitrogen levels have risen in surface and groundwater sources, resulting in elevated levels in drinking water supplies[57]. Untreated wastewater discharge has also contributed to the nitrate pollution of water resources.

Nitrate absorption is most often associated with the "blue baby syndrome" (methaemoglobinaemia). Infants under six months of age are particularly vulnerable to high levels of nitrates in drinking water. This is because nitrite (nitrate reduces to nitrite once entering into a human body) interferes with the blood's ability to carry oxygen to the body tissues, resulting in a bluish colour of a baby's skin. Levels higher than 10 milligrams of N/litre (US Standard) can have toxic effects on infants. Adults and older children are able to withstand much higher levels with no risk of methaemoglobinaemia[58].

Excessive nitrates in rivers and lakes cause eutrophication in many regions of the world, which disrupts aquatic ecosystems through oversupply of nutrients that cause the mass growth of algae and plants. This process eventually depletes most oxygen in the water and kills the aquatic organisms, rendering the water body lifeless and sterile.

Arsenic and fluoride

Some dangerous chemicals also occur naturally in groundwater, notably arsenic and fluoride. In Bangladesh, high concentrations of arsenic have been found in tube wells in 61 out of 64 districts[59]. Excessive arsenic levels in groundwater are also found in some parts of Argentina, Cambodia, Canada, Chile, China, India, Japan, Mexico, Philippines, Viet Nam and the United States.

Arsenic can cause severe and irreversible health effects – even in very small amounts. Early symptoms can range from the development of dark spots on the skin to a hardening of the skin into nodules, often on the palms and soles. Over time, the symptoms can become more pronounced and in some cases internal organs including the liver, kidneys and lungs can be affected[60]. In the most severe cases, cancer can occur in the skin and internal organs and limbs can be affected by gangrene. The damage due to arsenicosis in humans is irreversible. There is a need to know much more about the health impacts of chronic and relatively low levels of exposures to arsenic.

Another problem is high levels of fluoride in some groundwater sources. Although fluoride is found in all waters at some concentration, high fluoride concentrations are found mostly in calcium-deficient ground waters in certain geographical belts, such as one along the East Africa Rift and another from Turkey through Iraq, Iran, Afghanistan, India, northern Thailand and China[61]. With large populations in developing countries directly consuming groundwater, excessive levels of fluoride in groundwater pose serious health concerns. These range from dental fluorosis (discoloured, blackened or mottled teeth) to crippling skeletal fluorosis (permanent spine, bone and joint deformations). As with arsenicosis, the damage caused by fluorosis is irreversible.

Although the total number of people at risk with fluoride is not known, a conservative estimate would number in the tens of millions. In India, 16 of its 32 states have been identified as endemic for fluorosis[62]. Fluorosis is prevalent in large parts of China, and is caused not only by drinking fluoride in groundwater, but also by breathing airborne fluoride released from the burning of fluoride-laden coal[63]. In fluoride-affected rural areas in these countries, children with dental fluorosis are a common sight, as are severely crippled adults, illustrating the disabling effect of chronic exposure to excessive fluoride.

Radiation

Radiation is another type of pollution that causes adverse health effects in children. Examples of exposure to ionizing radiation include the Chernobyl nuclear power plant accident in 1986 and the use of radioactive materials during war. Depleted uranium, a weak radioactive material, is sometimes used as the heads of rounds fired from aircraft. During the Kosovo conflict in 1999, about 31,000 depleted uranium rounds were fired at targets on the ground[64]. Fact-finding missions by UNEP and WHO looked at the environmental and health impacts, respectively, of the use of depleted uranium in the conflict. Although the missions found no convincing evidence to indicate any health impact to people in Kosovo, it was noted that people could come into contact with depleted uranium by picking up objects from the ground. Naturally, children may be particularly at risk from exposure to depleted uranium because of their curiosity and lack of knowledge about the contamination.

Overexposure to ionising radiation, such as from nuclear fuels and radioactive isotopes used in medical facilities, can induce cancers, birth deformities and psychiatric disorders[65]. Studies of the health impacts of Chernobyl have associated a sharp increase in the incidences of childhood thyroid cancer with the accident[66]. The investigation of brain damage in utero found evidence suggesting retarded mental development and deviations in behavioural and emotional reactions in children who had been exposed[67].

Overexposure to ionising radiation, such as from nuclear fuels and radioactive isotopes used in medical facilities, can induce cancers, birth deformities and psychiatric disorders.

Radioactive pollution also includes radiation from non-ionising electromagnetic fields, such as radio waves and microwaves. Knowledge of the potential health effects of chronic and low exposure to electromagnetic fields is extremely limited. For example, some epidemiological studies have suggested an increased risk of leukaemia in children living near power lines. Whether this is due to exposure to extremely low frequency magnetic fields or some other factors in the environment has not been determined[68]. A recent study has suggested that exposure to radio frequency fields increases the incidence of lymphomas in genetically manipulated mice, but until at least two more large studies are conducted, the issues raised by that study cannot be fully answered[69]. Most known adverse health effects related to electromagnetic fields occur from exposure to radio frequency fields between one MHz and 10 GHz inducing heating in the body. Induced heating may adversely affect the development of a foetus[70].

Selected facts

- About 50 million people work on plantations in developing countries and are in direct contact with pesticides, while over 500 million more are exposed through other forms of agriculture[71]. In Egypt, over 1 million children between the ages of seven and 12 are hired by the agricultural cooperatives to take part in cotton pest management and are at risk of pesticide exposure[72].
- About 78 per cent of all gasoline sold in the world is unleaded and this will likely rise to over 84 per cent by 2005[73].
- Toxic poisoning in children accounts for about two per cent of all deaths by injury in children in developed countries and about five per cent in developing countries[74].
- In the Philippines, mining waste leaching into bays, streams, or lakes presents a serious concern. One mine dumped 40 billion tonnes of mining wastes into the ocean, just offshore, which resulted in elevated mercury levels in fish 100 miles away[75]. In the Amazon River basin, at least 130 tons of mercury is released into the environment every year from gold-mining activities at more than 2,000 mining sites using mercury amalgamation[76].

Taking action

- Communities and their governments worldwide should phase out the use of certain toxic chemicals, such as lead in gasoline and paint and the pesticides already banned in industrialized countries but still used in developing countries.
- Local communities and their local and national governments should recognize, evaluate and act with urgency to protect children from the effects of chemicals that are present in the environment. This applies to all countries, but especially to those in the developing world and in Eastern

Europe and countries of the former Soviet Union. In those countries the health impact of toxic exposures can be magnified by the unsafe use of chemicals, the lack of awareness about chemical risks and the effects of pollutants, and by an interaction among toxins, malnutrition and infectious diseases.

- Academic institutes, research laboratories and universities should expand toxicological studies to take into account synergistic and multiple effects of pollutants. They should also expand the existing bank of research on the specific toxicological effects on children in order to set safety limits and guidelines on a child's vulnerabilities rather than the current 'average adult' who is well nourished and healthy.
- Health-related research should be supported and assessments carried out to determine the health impacts of specific chemicals. The international community recently requested UNEP to undertake a global study of the health and environmental impacts of mercury. Among other things this study will undertake an assessment of the cost effectiveness of current mercury anti-pollution measures and technologies.
- Communities and their local and national governments should promote the development and use of clean energy sources whenever possible.

Examples of what works

- In December 2000, over 100 countries agreed to regulate the production, import, export, disposal and use of 12 Persistent Organic Pollutants (POP) – including DDT, polychlorinated biphenyls, dioxins and furans. Most of the 12 chemicals are subject to an immediate ban, with the exception of an exemption for DDT when it is used to control mosquitoes. The Convention on POPs was formally adopted and signed by ministers and other government representatives at a diplomatic conference in May 2001 in Stockholm and will enter into force when 50 Governments have signed and ratified it.

- As a result of the phasing out of lead additives in gasoline, which was part of the agreement reached in the Partnership for Pollution Prevention at the 1994 Summit of the Americas, the average gasoline lead content in North America is now among the lowest in the world[77]. In the United States emissions of lead have decreased nearly 90 per cent over the last 20 years, mainly due to the phasing out of leaded gasoline. A parallel decline in blood-lead levels accompanied the phase-out of leaded gasoline and the introduction of catalytic converters in 1973[78].
- Extensive clean-up activities have recently begun in Ethiopia, where the UN Food and Agriculture Organization (FAO) estimates there is the largest build-up of obsolete pesticides in Africa. Nearly 3,000 tons of obsolete pesticides stored throughout the country could be leaking into the soil, polluting water supplies, and threatening the health of thousands of people[79].
- More than 1 million people in Latin America, including women and children, are involved in small-scale gold mining, which involves the use of mercury. With international support, a local NGO in Venezuela introduced an alternative mining technology, which uses less mercury and can increase gold recovery, to Bolivar's Caroni River region. Gold miners participating in the project received practical information and medical advice, in addition to learning the technique, and continued mining with reduced hazards and boosted production[80].

Indoor and Outdoor Air Pollution

Air pollution – both indoor and outdoor – is a major environment-related health threat, causing a range of respiratory and cardiovascular ailments. Unhealthy air is breathed by an estimated 1.1 billion people and claims 3 million lives a year[81].

Table 4: Examples of chemical pollutants

Chemicals found in food and water	Chemicals found in the home and workplace	Chemicals found outdoors
▪ Lead ▪ Deliberate or accidental food adulteration ▪ Nitrates in drinking water ▪ Aflatoxin and other natural food toxicants ▪ Trace pesticides in water supply, many from agro-chemicals ▪ High mineral content in drinking water ▪ Aluminium ▪ Arsenic in groundwater ▪ Fluoride in groundwater ▪ Copper ▪ Mercury in fish ▪ PCBs/dioxins in food	▪ Carbon monoxide from combustion of fossil fuels ▪ Lead from paint ▪ Tobacco smoke ▪ Asbestos ▪ Smoke from combustion of coal, wood or other biomass fuels ▪ Insecticides and herbicides used around the home ▪ Mercury ▪ Radon ▪ Formaldehyde from insulation	▪ Lead from automobile exhausts and external paint ▪ Sulfur dioxide and oxides of nitrogen from industries, power stations and auto engines ▪ Ozone and photochemical smog ▪ Carbon monoxide from combustion of fuels ▪ Cadmium, mercury compounds and other heavy metals ▪ Dioxins, PCBs and pesticides ▪ Agricultural chemicals

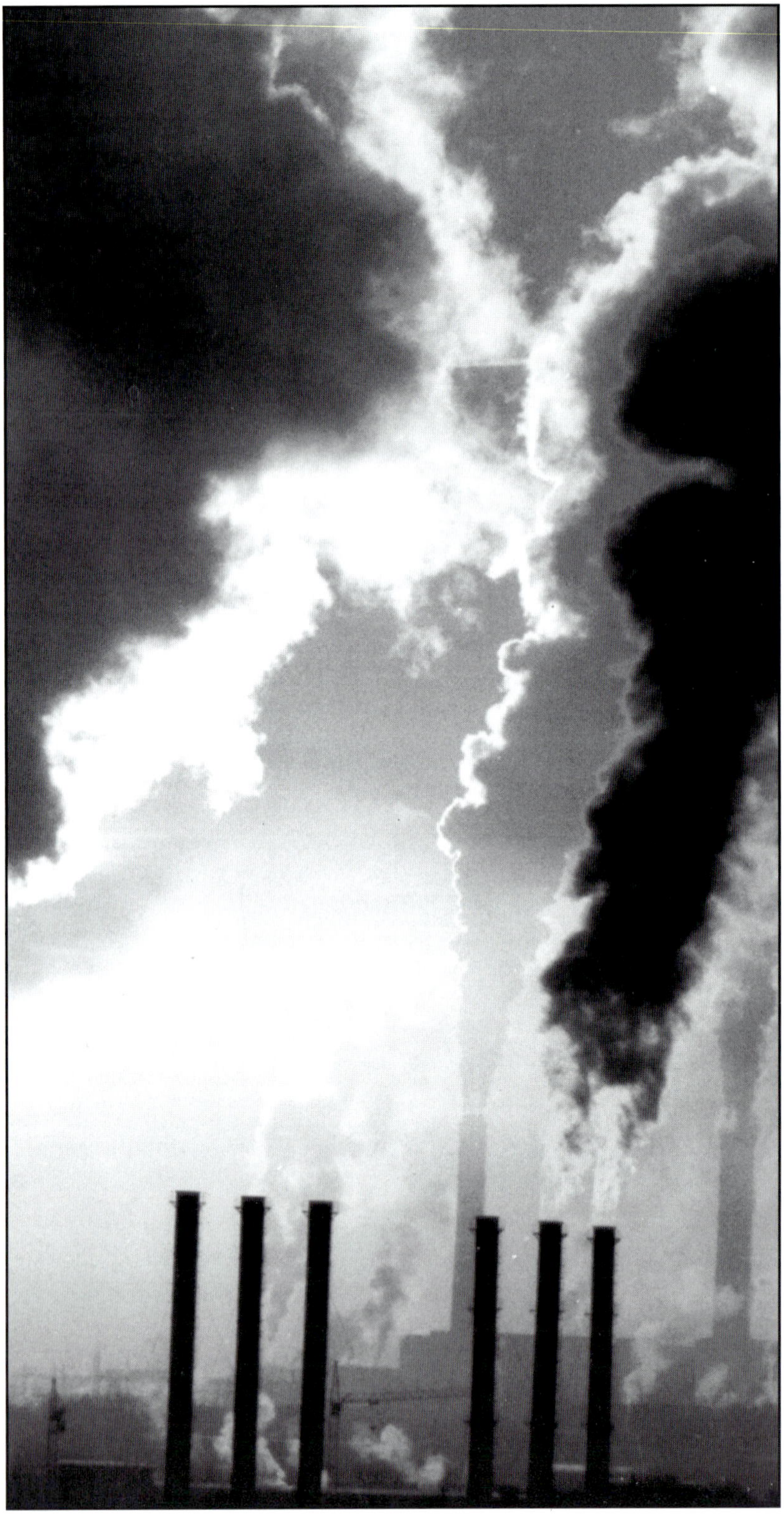

Air pollution – both indoor and outdoor – is a major environment-related health threat, causing a range of respiratory and cardiovascular ailments.

Indoor air pollution

Indoor air pollution occurs when fossil or biomass fuels are used for cooking and heating in crowded and poorly ventilated settings. Of all forms of air pollution worldwide, indoor air pollution from open fires or inefficient stoves is the single greatest cause of ill-health[82].

About 2.5 billion people are dependant on biomass fuel for cooking and heating, of whom 75 per cent are in developing countries[83]. Of this 2.5 billion population, approximately 800 million depend on agricultural residues and animal dung as sources of fuel due to severe fuel wood shortage[84].

These people often use low-efficiency, smoky cooking stoves. For example, the efficiency of the three-stone fire traditionally used in many developing countries is only about 10 to 15 per cent. The cooking stoves produce heavy smoke with fine particles, carbon monoxide and carcinogenic compounds such as polycyclic aromatic hydrocarbons (PAHs)[85]. Measurements of indoor particle concentration in rural households of developing countries greatly exceeded the 1987 WHO recognized guideline values and air quality standards used in the United States and Europe[89], typically by some 20 times higher[87].

Indoor air contamination is also caused by biological particles, such as pollen, mould, the droppings of mites, insects, microorganisms, as well as the non-biological particles, such as lead, carbon monoxide, asbestos and synthetic chemicals. Women and children, who spend the most time indoors, are the prime victims of the resulting indoor air pollution. These dust particles contain irritants and infectious agents that can cause or worsen ARI. Another very important source of indoor air pollution is tobacco smoke.

Outdoor air pollution

Outdoor air pollution is a particularly serious threat to the swelling populations of the world's cities. With the increased combustion of fossil fuels, industrial processes and growing car use, urban populations are exposed to a long list of pollutants that include sulphur dioxide, nitrogen oxide, nitrogen dioxide, carbon monoxide, ozone, lead, dioxins, suspended particulate matter and a host of volatile organic compounds. Open burning of urban waste with high components of plastics like polyvinyl chloride (PVC) is also a significant source of dioxins, furans and heavy metals in many communities. People who are poor often live close to these sites or work in them.

Cities in developing countries have much higher average pollutant concentrations than cities in industrialized countries (see figure 6). In the late 1990s, the average annual concentration of PM10 (small particles with diameters less than 10 microns) in North American, Western European and Japanese cities ranged from 30 to 45 micrograms per cubic metre. Chinese and Indian cities, on the other hand, had averages of nearly 200 micrograms per cubic metre of PM10[89].

Children are most susceptible to air pollutants in the first month of life.

In addition, forest fires, whether accidental or started to clear forestland for agricultural purposes, have been the cause of severe smoke haze pollution in Asia, Latin America and North America – causing serious health concerns for children and the elderly. In addition, dust storms in many regions of the world (especially in Central Asia), the magnitude of which is aggravated by desertification and deforestation, represent another significant source of outdoor air pollution.

Impact of air pollution on children

Children are most susceptible to air pollutants in the first month of life[88], particularly during episodes of severe pollution. Although the risk declines with each passing month, air pollutants remain a risk to children. The health effects of air pollution depend in large measure on the types of pollutants inhaled and the exposure level (i.e., frequency, concentration, etc.) of the child. Estimates suggest that up to 60 per cent of the global ARI burden of disease is associated with indoor air pollution and other environmental factors such as ambient air pollution and housing conditions[90]. Infants and young children, particularly girls, who are often requested to help their mothers in household chores, are most at risk.

Infants are exposed to pollutants while resting on the backs of their mothers as they tend fires. Girls are exposed as they assume their share of household cooking. In India, respiratory infections linked to solid fuel use are estimated to cause 290,000-440,000 premature deaths a year in children under five years of age[91]. The small particles in polluted air enter deep into the lungs and respiratory organs, causing viral and bacterial ARI, the most severe being pneumonia. ARI account for 67 per cent of deaths in the world's children from birth to 14 years[92]. Irritation that would not significantly affect adults may result in more severe obstruction and damage in a child's lungs since they are still forming and are more vulnerable. Childhood ARI-related death rates are high even in nations where the infant mortality rates are low. In high-

FIGURE 6: AIR POLLUTION IN CITIES OF DEVELOPING COUNTRIES

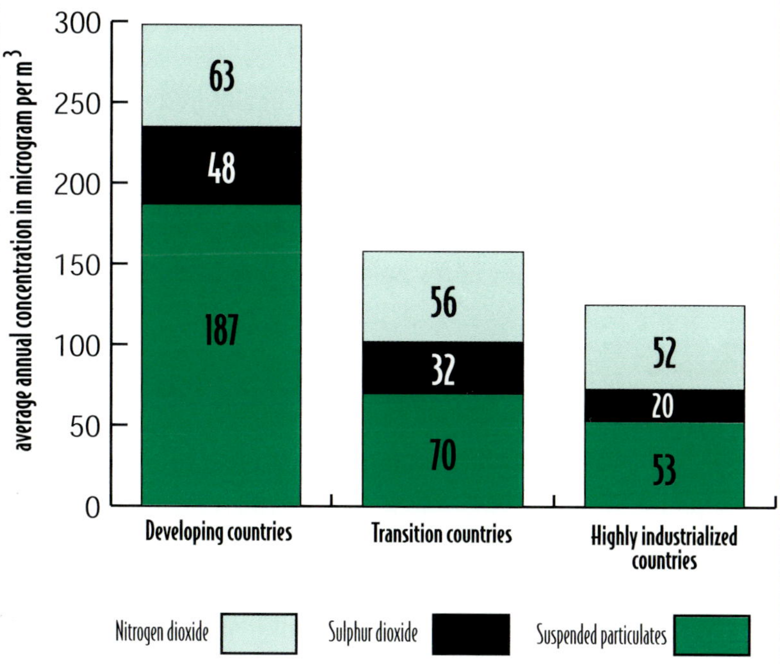

Source: United Nations Centre for Human Settlements (Habitat), The State of the World's Cities 2001, UNCHS (Habitat) Publication Unit, Nairobi, 2001

Adults who smoke can also put children at risk for tobacco-related illnesses.

income countries, ARI is the third leading cause of death in children under four. In developing countries over 64 million cases of ARI are reported per year[93].

Indoor air pollution is not only linked to ARI. Studies in developing countries have linked exposure to indoor air pollution with chronic respiratory diseases such as asthma (see box 10), chronic obstructive pulmonary disease, lung cancer, stillbirths and low-birth weight[94]. Lung cancer has been found to result from long-term exposure to cooking with coal in China[95]. Outdoor air contamination can also cause pulmonary irritation, interfere with foetal growth and infant development, impair lung functions, exacerbate viral infections, bronchitis and pneumonia and worsen heart problems, asthma and emphysema.

Adults who smoke can also put children at risk for tobacco-related illnesses. Environmental tobacco smoke (ETS) has been linked to a number of serious health problems in children, including upper respiratory infections, chronic coughs, asthma, chronic ear infections and sudden infant death syndrome[96]. A 1997 study also connected ETS to abnormal cholesterol levels in children. It found that children who were exposed to environmental tobacco smoke at home had high-density lipoprotein cholesterol levels – the so called "good" cholesterol - as much as 10 per cent lower than the levels of children who came from non smoking households[97].

Selected facts

- Sixty per cent of deaths caused by acute respiratory infections (ARI) occur in children under 15 years of age, mainly in low and middle-income countries. Globally, this amounts to an estimated 2 million deaths among children and to over 64 million reported cases of ARI. It is the second leading cause of disease for children under four years of age in these countries[99].
- Outdoor air pollution causes more than 50,000 premature deaths and 400,000 new cases of chronic bronchitis per year in 11 East Asian cities alone[100].

Box 10: Asthma

In developed countries, asthma is the leading chronic disease among children. In the United States alone, it affects 4.8 million children under the age of 18 and asthma-related hospitalization and death rates are increasing.

Air pollution, both indoor and outdoor, is one of the triggers for asthma episodes. A recent study was able to associate high concentrations of ozone in the air with the development of asthma in children exercising outdoors[98].

Indoor air pollution in developed countries can be attributed to factors such as:

- Increased use of household chemicals;
- Use of synthetic building and furnishing materials;
- Increased insulation and decreased ventilation; and
- Tobacco smoke.

Sources: Morain, Claudia et al., "Understanding Asthma", Health Management Bulletin-Information for Asthma Patients and Their Friends, American Medical Association (Division of Clinical Immunology & Allergy, Children's Hospital), Los Angeles, 1997.

- It has been estimated by the World Bank, which is providing technical assistance to Bangladesh to cut lead poisoning, that the country could avoid 15,000 deaths and save $200 million to $800 million annually by reducing air pollution in the cities of Dhaka, Cittagong, Rajshehi and Kluna[101].
- In the United States, the number of children with asthma has doubled in the past 15 years and there is now an estimated one in 15 children under age 18 who has asthma[102].
- As a result of forest fires in Indonesia in 1997-98 it is generally believed that the health of approximately 20 million

people in the region was adversely affected by the smoke, particularly through upper respiratory tract infections and asthma. Skin and eye diseases were also prevalent[103].

- In some parts of Europe and Central Asia, the concentrations of nitrogen oxides and particulate matter are up to three times higher than the WHO recommended levels[104].
- In 1994 it was estimated that in developing countries, over 80 per cent of children from urban areas between the ages of three and five years of age and 100 per cent under two had average blood levels of lead exceeding the threshold of 10 µg /dl set by the U.S. Centers for Disease Control and Prevention[105].

Taking action

- Air pollution control regulations should be enforced in cities, especially phasing out leaded gasoline, controlling pollution from coal-fired boilers and substituting cleaner or renewable energy for fossil fuels.
- Sustainable energy use should be promoted to alleviate energy problems in rural and urban developing areas, such as dissemination of improved cooking stoves, development of alternative, environmentally sound household energy sources, improvement of kitchen ventilation and community forestry.
- Environmental management strategies should be combined with improved nutrition, clean water, adequate sanitation, prenatal health care, immunization programmes and early childhood care programmes. These measures will help prevent low birth weight, strengthen children's natural defence mechanisms and help protect them from illnesses and disease.
- More research should be conducted to better understand the relationship between childhood illness and air pollution, in order to formulate integrated health and environment approaches, which reduce childhood exposure to air

pollutants. ARI, particularly pneumonia in young children, can be reduced effectively by environmental and nutritional improvements.

Examples of what works

- The most successful sustainable energy projects in the field are those that support greater income-generating projects and economic opportunities, mainly for women. For example, in Mali, a recent project trained women's groups to operate diesel generators as formal businesses. They became energy entrepreneurs, selling energy, which in turn increased economic activity in the community[106].
- Cars using alternative energies are being developed and are now being introduced to the mass market. Electric, hybrid electric, compressed natural gas and fuel cell vehicles are likely to be available to consumers in the near future[107].
- Alternative cooking stoves that are more energy efficient and promote a shift from using traditional fuels (wood and charcoal) and significantly reduce exposure to indoor air pollution must be encouraged. In areas where these stoves are not yet available, some community leaders are promoting the use of a cooking window or a chimney as a way of evacuating smoke from the cooking area.

Cars using alternative energies are being developed and are now being introduced to the mass market.

Natural Resource Degradation

Currently, there is enough food to feed the world; yet, 149 million children are still malnourished[108]. A nutritionally adequate diet for the world's rapidly growing population will necessitate tripling food production over the next 50 years[109]. This task will be an enormous challenge in the face of growing environmental degradation and contamination – two factors that often compromise household food security and health, especially for children.

Land degradation

The distribution of fertile soils and favourable growing conditions does not match that of the world's population. Global projections for food supplies by region suggest that future problems will be mainly concentrated in sub-Saharan Africa and South Asia[110]. The worldwide loss of arable land is exacerbated by land and natural resource degradation caused by a series of processes and human activities, such as deforestation, desertification, soil erosion, over grazing, over-use of fertilisers and pesticides, lack of watershed management, excessive withdrawal of groundwater, pollution, poor land-use planning and uncontrolled dumping of wastes. Moreover, the rising demand for meat, fish, poultry and dairy products encourages farmers to raise livestock, displacing subsistence food crops for growing fodder and feed crops for animals, hence, making less efficient use of the land[111].

Currently, there is enough food to feed the world; yet, 149 million children are still malnourished.

Fisheries

Nearly 1 billion people depend on fish as their primary source of protein[112]. For them, increasingly difficult times lie ahead. The degradation of coastal marine environments, the modification and destruction of habitats, over-fishing and pollution have compounded the overexploitation of an estimated 70 per cent of marine fisheries (see figure 7), causing catastrophic reductions of annual harvests for local fishing communities throughout the world.

Selected facts

- Nearly 30 per cent of the world's population suffers from one or more of the multiple forms of malnutrition[113].
- 149 million children are malnourished, two thirds of them in Asia. The absolute number of malnourished children has increased in Africa[114].
- In Africa, only North Africa has been able to make major increases in the per capita calorie supply. Land degradation

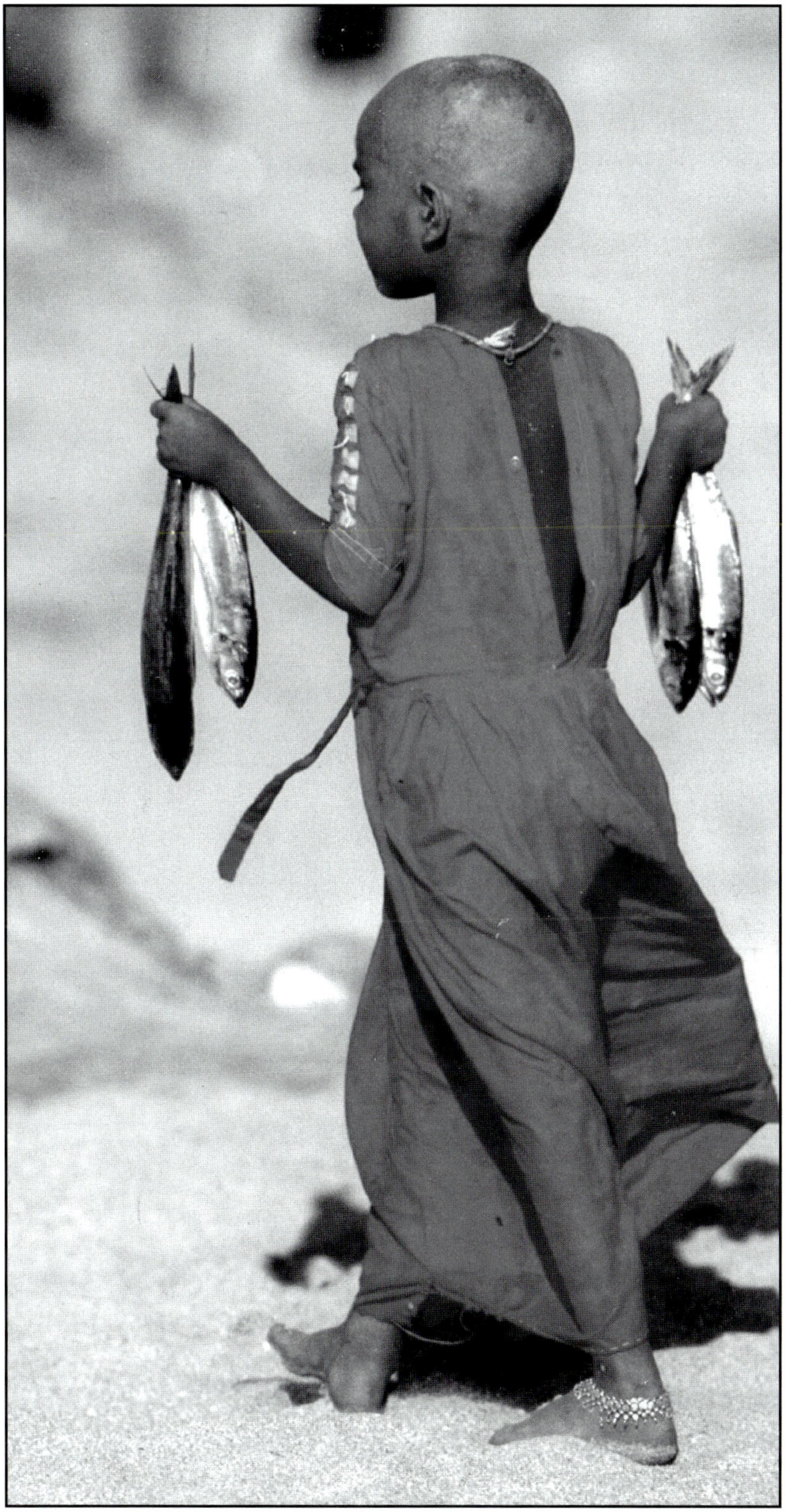

Nearly 1 billion people depend on fish as their primary source of protein.

Figure 7: Marine fisheries

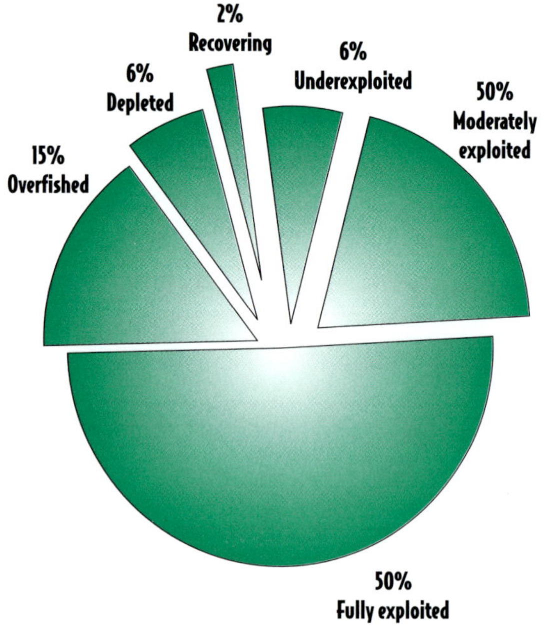

Source: Food and Agriculture Organization at http://www.unep.ch/earthw/em17.htm

and drought are important causes of the decline in southern Africa[115].

- Roundworm, whipworm and hookworm (helminth diseases) affect about 400 million school-age children throughout the world[116].

Impacts of natural resource degradation

Millions of children under five die each year in developing countries mainly from preventable diseases. It is estimated that half of these deaths are either directly or indirectly attributable to malnutrition[117]. Foetal development also hinges on the mother's nutritional status. Under-nutrition during pregnancy and in early childhood can adversely affect physical and behavioural development, with short- and long-term consequences (see figure 8). Maternal anaemia (iron deficiency), which is often linked to protein energy deficiency, renders the mother more vulnerable to diseases and increases her chances of giving birth to lower birth-weight babies. Low birth-weight babies are vulnerable and more likely to die at an early age or face severe physical and developmental problems during infancy and beyond. Land degradation and natural resource depletion can contribute to malnutrition.

Millions of children under five die each year in developing countries mainly from preventable diseases.

Malnourished children can be listless and have slow social and cognitive development, which can lead to poor school performance and disadvantages in later adult life. Furthermore, childhood micronutrient deficiency (vitamin A, iron) can retard child growth, increase the duration and severity of illness and render children more sensitive to toxic agents at lower levels.

FIGURE 8: CONSEQUENCES OF MALNUTRITION AND ITS INTERGENERATIONAL CYCLE

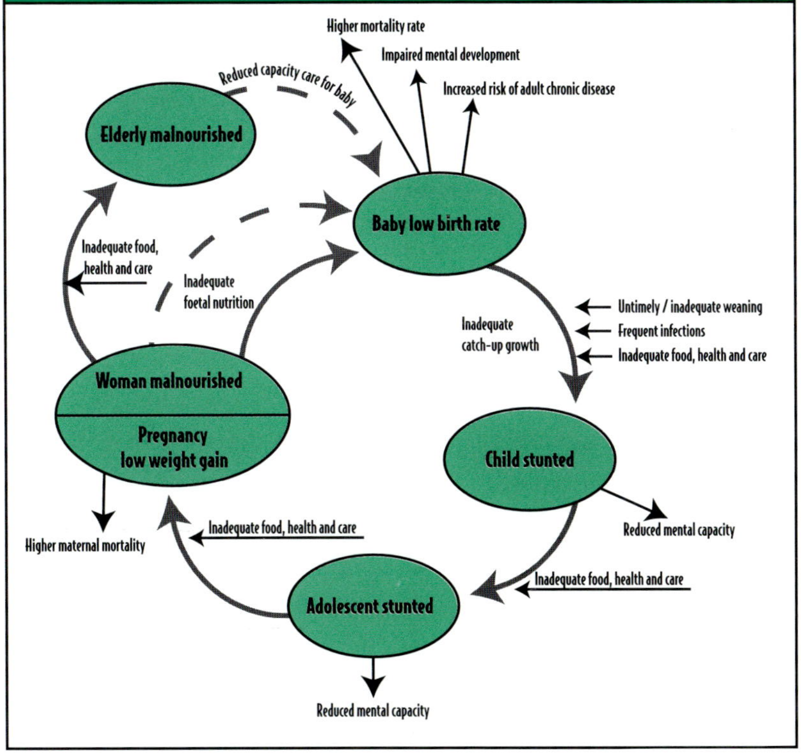

Source: Administrative Committee on Coordination / Sub-commitee on Nutrition (ACC/SCN) (2000); Low Birthweight: report of a meeting in Dhaka, Bangladesh on 14-17 June 1999. Eds. Pojda J. and Kelly L. Nutrition Policy Paper #18, Geneva, 2000.

Research suggests that child growth can be harmed in unhygienic surroundings even before acute infections occur. It is believed that early childhood nutritional deficits coupled with an unsanitary environment lead to impaired growth and a failure to maximize genetic potential. Even if a child is not obviously sick, an unclean environment poses a constant threat to the immune system. Nutrients from food that should help a child to grow are instead used by the body to support its immune system, thus impairing growth.

A hungry child is a weak child. A weak child is a sick child. Frequent illness will almost surely result in physical weakness and nutritional deficiency. Consequently, poor nutritional status further weakens a child's immune system, making the child all the more susceptible to diseases and pollutants. For example, frequent and prolonged diarrhoea episodes are important contributors to malnutrition and malnutrition increases susceptibility to more severe diarrhoea, and, in turn, increases the likelihood of death due to this ailment[118]. The cycle of "malnutrition ➔ infection ➔ malnutrition" (see figure 9) pushes children down the spiral of poor growth and early death. This vicious spiral can, to a large extent, be prevented. Environmental management strategies can have an important contribution to make in this regard.

Moreover, the amount of energy and time spent by women and children, especially girls, collecting water, fuel and fodder is proportional to the abundance of natural resources. Often, girls will be forced to abandon school in order to meet their family's needs for these resources. All in all, environmental degradation intensifies the drudgery of women and children, further undermining their health and nutritional status.

Helminth diseases

The contamination of land and vegetables along with poor sanitation and hygiene is associated with another important problem for children – helminth diseases. Hundreds of millions of school-age children throughout the developing world are currently infected by roundworm, whipworm and/or hookworm, which cause helminth infections. Coming into contact with soil or vegetables that contain the eggs or young worms of these parasites infects children. The highest rates of roundworm and whipworm infections are found in the groups five to nine and 10 to 14 years old[119].

Worms consume the nutrients from the children they infect. Hence, the infected children are robbed of nutrients needed for their young bodies to grow, which, in turn, triggers or aggravates malnutrition, retards physical development, and stunts growth. These parasites destroy the tissues and organs they live in, causing pain and various health problems. Roundworms cause structural problems in the small intestine in children and also cause serious pulmonary disease in children. Severe whipworm infections are associated with high incidence of dysentery, chronic colitis, anaemia and growth retardation. Hookworm infections cause iron deficiency anaemia and may result in minor infections developing into severe anaemia in children and adolescent girls[120].

Taking action

- Communities and governments should strengthen support to programmes that reinforce local food systems, where possible, through measures to combat desertification. They should promote sustainable agricultural practices, water resource management and integrated pest management to minimise artificial pesticide use, encourage rural and urban kitchen gardens and give favourable economic incentives to farmers and low-income households (such as micro-credits).
- Communities and governments should alleviate the impacts of environmental degradation on women and children. An example of how this could be done is through supporting or strengthening water supply, agro- and social forestry, household energy and fuel-efficient stove projects. The participatory role of the community should be strengthened.

Figure 9: The most vulnerable

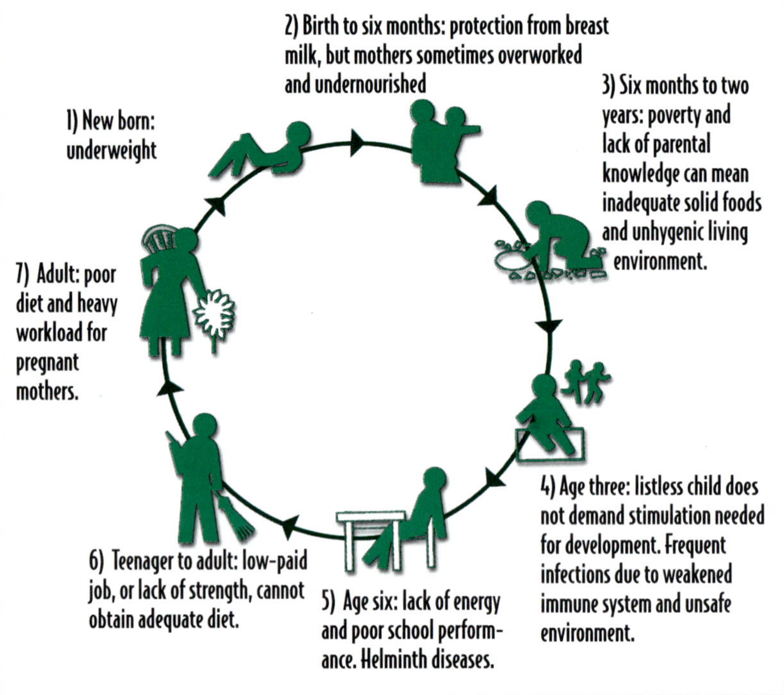

Source: Adapted from United Nations Environment Programme and United Nations Children's Fund, The State of the Environment 1990: Children and the Environment, UNEP and UNICEF, New York, 1990.

- Individuals and families can prevent helminth infections through proper management of human faeces and good hygiene so as not to pollute the ground or drinking water at the source and in the home.
- Individuals and their communities can promote health and hygiene education in schools.
- Schools should provide safe water and sanitary facilities to break the worm transmission routes.
- Three basic interventions are known to reduce helminth infections: for achieving sustainable results, drug treatment should be provided in combination with sanitary improvement and health education.

Examples of what works

- Fifty per cent of the women and children of Bangladesh suffer from vitamin A deficiency – a condition that has been linked to growth retardation, blindness, increased susceptibility to infections, and sometimes death. It also increases the risk of maternal-infant transmission among HIV-positive women. To address this challenge, a community organization developed a home gardening assistance programme to promote year-round gardening and the diversification of fruit and vegetable varieties that are rich in vitamin A. This programme has also increased overall food intake of the targeted families and provided them with extra income from selling part of their fruit and vegetable production[121].
- In the Mysore District of Karnataka, India, most families are landless or small-land holders. With international support, a local NGO initiated a small project in 1991 to promote reforestation and horticulture. By 1999 the participating 100 families had substantially improved their livelihoods with diverse, ecologically sound activities, including developing vegetable gardens and mango and cashew orchards. They also are composting, growing tuber crops under the trees and processing and marketing their products in local markets. As a result, children in this community are better nourished and are enjoying a cleaner environment[122].
- The Indian farmers of Oaxaca, Mexico have been producing coffee for more than 120 years. In 1984, 17 communities wanted to break free from corporate intermediaries and the persistent side effects of the pesticides. They formed an organization, called the Union of Indian Communities of the Isthmus Region (UCIRI), and elected to produce their coffee organically. Today, international inspections take place twice a year and the group is exporting its organic coffee to several European countries, Canada, the United States and Japan. More than 250 organizations of small farmers are involved and more than

3,500 families have tripled their income (from a yearly income of US$ 280 in 1983 to US$ 860 in 1999). They have a higher yield of coffee, corn and bean production by means of organic management. Furthermore, UCIRI has initiated health care services, cooperative stores, improved housing, and built a training facility that educates young people from around the country in organic farming methodologies. The model has been documented and is now being replicated in other areas of the country, including Chiapas, Guerrero and Puebla. The entire project was done without any donations, only credit[123].

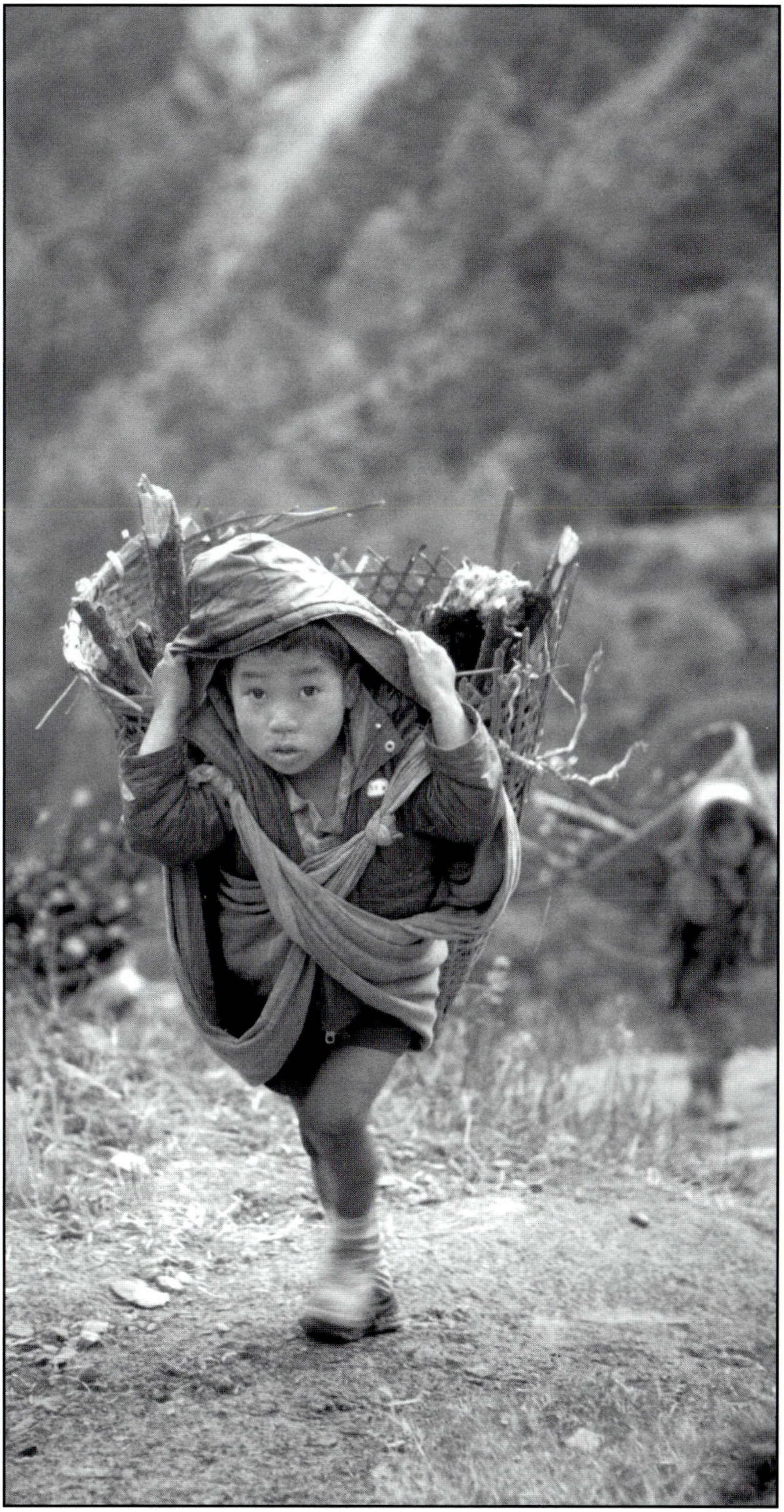

Environmental degradation intensifies the drudgery of women and children, further undermining their health and nutritional status.

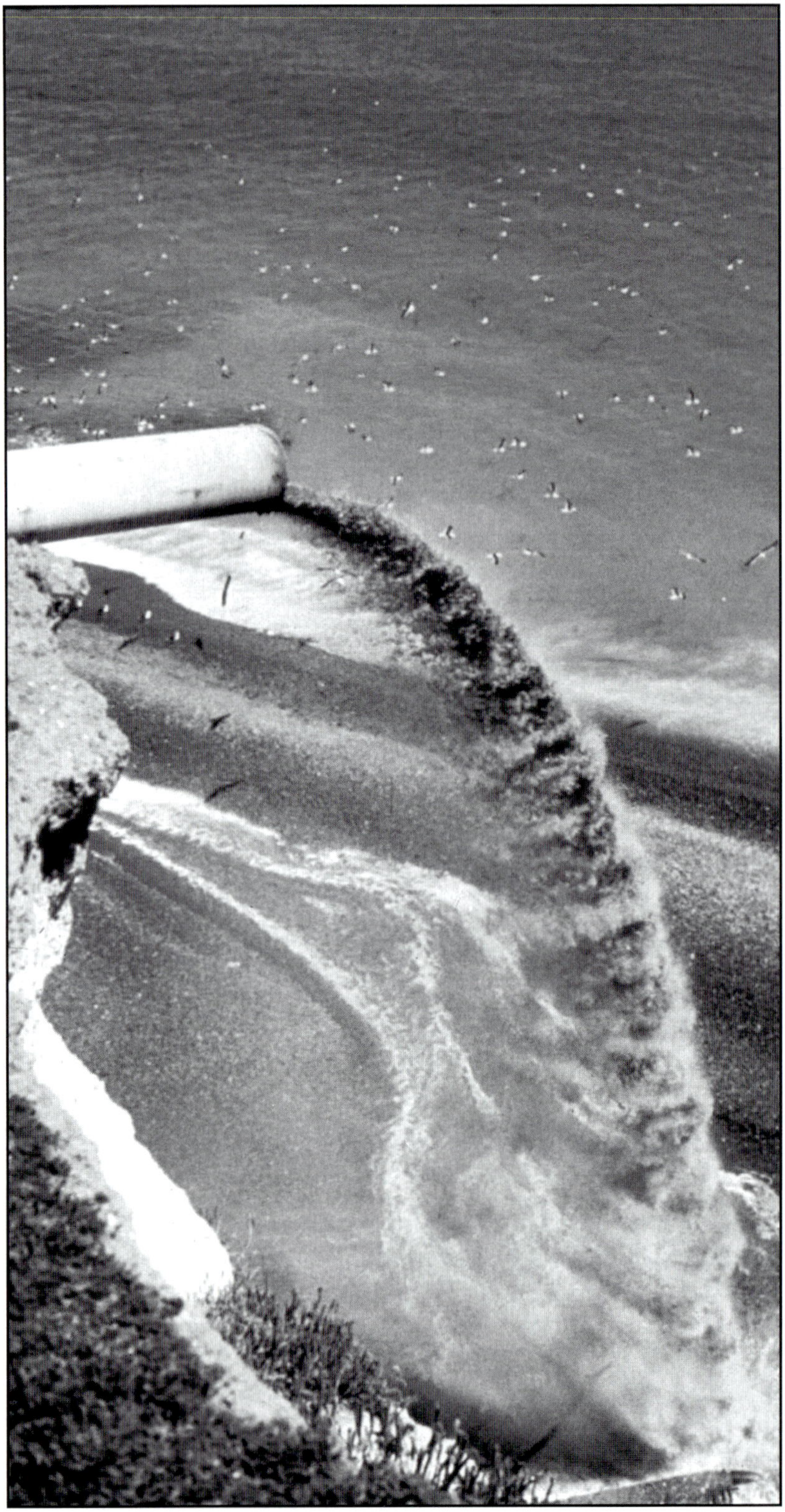

Global environmental challenges require concerted responses on the part of the international community.

4 Global Environmental Problems

At the dawn of the third millennium, a powerful and complex web of interactions is contributing to unprecedented global trends in environmental degradation. These forces include rapid globalization and urbanization, pervasive poverty, unsustainable consumption patterns and population growth. Often serving to compound the effects and intensity of the environmental problems described in the previous section, global environmental challenges require concerted responses on the part of the international community. Global climate change, the depletion of the ozone layer, desertification, deforestation, the loss of the planet's biological diversity and the transboundary movements of hazardous wastes and chemicals are all environmental problems that touch every nation and adversely affect the lives and health of their populations. As with other environment-related challenges, children are disproportionately vulnerable to and suffer most from the effects of these global trends.

Moreover, all of these global environmental trends have long-term effects on people and societies and are either difficult or impossible to reverse over the period of one generation. Unless effective global actions are taken early, we will end up plundering our children's heritage and future in an unprecedented way. This chapter describes five major global environmental problems and points to the potential impact on children and future generations.

The repercussions of climate change will disproportionately affect those who are least able to adapt – the poor and the most vulnerable sections of society, including children.

Climate Change

It is now widely recognized that global warming over the past 50 years is largely due to human activities that have released greenhouse gases into the atmosphere. The most recent assessment report by the Intergovernmental Panel on Climate Change (IPCC) concludes that the global average surface temperature has increased by about 0.6°C during the 20th century.

The seemingly small rise of mean temperature is already showing adverse effects. One of the consequences has been a rise in the global average sea level[1]. Another effect has been more frequent and intensified droughts in recent decades in parts of Asia and Africa. Additionally, in most mid and high latitudes of the Northern Hemisphere continents, precipitation has increased by 0.5 to 1.0 per cent per decade in the 20th century[2].

The world's emissions of greenhouse gases, notably carbon dioxide, continue to increase. The most recent estimates are that atmospheric concentrations of the greenhouse gas carbon dioxide (CO2) will double or triple pre-industrial levels by the end of this century. As a result, global surface temperature is expected to increase by 1.4 to 5.8 degrees Celsius from 1990 to 2100[3].

The repercussions of climate change will disproportionately affect those who are least able to adapt – the poor and the most vulnerable sections of society, including children. For example, scientists project that this level of warming could, among other things:

- Greatly exacerbate the range, frequency and intensity of natural disasters, from flooding, to droughts, to torrential rains, ice-storms, tornadoes and hurricanes;

- Cause sea levels to rise by between nine and 80 centimetres by 2100[4], due to the expansion of warming waters and the melting of polar icecaps and other glaciers, which in turn may produce deadly flooding in many low-lying areas and small island States, displacing millions from their homes;
- Increase the number of environmental refugees resulting from weather-related disasters;
- Augment the risk of disease migration and disease outbreaks; and
- Render large areas of the world "uninsurable" due to the magnitude of property damage from disasters.

It is widely recognized that climate change, by altering local weather patterns and by disturbing life-supporting natural systems and processes, has significant implications for human health. While the range of health effects is diverse, often unpredictable in magnitude, and sometimes slow to emerge, children remain among the most vulnerable to these threats.

Higher temperatures, heavier rainfall, and changes in climate variability would encourage vectors of some infectious diseases (such as malaria, schistosomiasis, dengue fever, yellow fever and encephalitis) to multiply and expand into new geographical regions, intensifying the already overwhelming threats to children from such diseases.

There is also evidence that El Niño – a vast natural climatic phenomenon that can bring intense floods and droughts in many parts of the globe – is becoming more frequent as a result of global warming and could further aggravate health problems in many parts of the world. Excessive flooding is, for example, a prime cause of cholera and other water-borne and food-borne infections to which children are particularly susceptible.

While heavy rains will become more frequent, there will also be more periods of drought and increased spreading of the deserts. Scientists predict that a lack of rain, warmer temperatures and increases in evaporation could have severe implications in terms of water availability and food security, reducing crop yields in Africa, further compromising child nutrition[5].

There are also numerous health effects, both in terms of disease and injury, associated with extreme weather events, such as heat waves, storms and floods. Extreme weather events can exacerbate health issues such as asthma and respiratory problems due to worsening air pollution, precisely those diseases that most significantly burden children.

Extreme weather events can excerbate health issues such as asthma and respiratory problems.

The international response to this issue is embodied in the 1992 United Nations Framework Convention on Climate Change (UNFCCC) and its 1997 Kyoto Protocol. The Convention sets principles and an agenda for action with the ultimate objective of stabilizing greenhouse gas emissions in the atmosphere at safe levels. It provides for: cooperation and exchange of information; leadership by industrialized countries in modifying long-term emission trends; financial and technological support for the efforts of developing countries; and responses to vulnerability. The UNFCCC has been in force since 1994 and, with over 180 countries having ratified it, is accepted nearly universally. On the other hand, while 80 countries have signed the Kyoto Protocol, which sets legally-binding emissions reduction targets for developed countries (5.2 per cent below 1990 levels on average in the period from 2008 to 2012), fewer than 50 countries have ratified it as this book goes to press. For the Kyoto Protocol to enter into force and become legally binding it has to be ratified by 55 countries, including those industrialized countries representing at least 55 per cent of the total 1990 carbon dioxide emissions from this group. However, of those countries that have currently ratified the Protocol, none are among the world's largest emitters.

Efforts are continuing to have the Kyoto Protocol enter into force as early as August 2002. Headway has been made, particularly following meetings in July 2001 in Bonn, Germany and November 2001 in Marrakesh, Morocco. Governments (with the US declining) agreed to detailed rules for the implementation of the Protocol, particularly on dealing with financial and technological support to developing countries, compliance, reporting, and the Protocol's implementing mechanisms, which include emissions trading, joint implementation, and investments in clean technologies in developing countries.

Ozone Layer Depletion

Ozone in the atmosphere's upper layer, the stratosphere, protects humans, animals and plants from the damaging effects of UV-B radiation from the sun. Without it, all life on earth would cease to exist. However, the use of chlorofluorocarbons (CFCs) and other ozone-depleting substances (ODS) are slowly eating away at the stratospheric ozone layer, creating a major potential health hazard. While the concentrations of ODS in the lower atmosphere peaked in about 1994 and is now slowly declining due to worldwide efforts to phase out the use of CFCs and other damaging substances, significant health threats relating to ozone depletion persist.

Past (and current) emissions of ODS result in increases of ultraviolet radiation reaching the Earth's surface which can pose several health effects[6]:

- Increase of melanoma and non-melanoma skin cancers;
- Cause or acceleration of eye cataracts development;
- Reduce effectiveness of the immune system;
- Impact on nutrition (e.g. reduced plant yield);
- Damage to ocean ecosystems and reduced fish yield (by killing microbial organisms in the ocean).

Skin cancer is the most worrisome health impact of ozone depletion. Overexposure to the sun's harmful ultraviolet (UV) light may damage children's skin. Recent studies indicate that excessive sunburns experienced by children 10 to 15 years of age increase by threefold the chance of developing malignant melanoma, the most deadly kind of skin cancer, later in life[7]. In Europe, evaluations of ultraviolet-related skin cancers suggest that, despite the decline in ODS concentrations, skin cancer incidences will not begin to fall until about 2060.

The international response to this issue is embodied in the Convention for the Protection of the Ozone Layer, which was concluded in Vienna in 1985. The Vienna Convention set an important precedent because nations for the first time agreed in principle to tackle a global environmental problem before its effects were felt. The Convention's 1987 Montreal Protocol on Substances that Deplete the Ozone Layer has been remarkably successful. Production of the most damaging ozone-depleting substances was eliminated, except for a few critical uses, by 1996 in developed countries and should be phased out by 2010 in developing countries. Thanks to these measures, it is currently estimated the CFC concentration in the ozone layer is expected to recover to pre-1980 levels by the year 2050.

Desertification

Desertification, resulting in part from deforestation, is a significant threat to the arid, semi-arid and dry sub-humid regions of the world – which account for 40 per cent of the Earth's land surface. Throughout the world, drylands still provide much of the world's food in the form of grain and livestock, yet close to 70 per cent of the world's drylands are degraded[8], thus diminishing the productive land per capita and decreasing food security. The most common forms of unsustainable land use are over-cultivation, overgrazing, deforestation and poor irrigation practices. These susceptible soils – mainly located in the savannahs of Africa, the Great Plains and the Pampas of the Americas, the Steppes of southeast Europe and Asia, the outback of Australia and the margins of the Mediterranean – are particularly vulnerable due to the fact that they recover very slowly from disturbances and further deteriorate due to rain and wind erosion and chemical and physical deterioration of the soil structure.

More than 250 million people are directly affected by desertification and 1 billion people in more than 100 countries are at risk[9]. These people include many of the world's poorest and most marginalized citizens. In Africa, land degradation is threatening economic and physical survival. Recurrent droughts increase soil degradation problems, which, in turn, magnify the effect of drought, both of which enhance the conditions that can cause widespread famines. The consequences of desertification include:

More than 250 million people are directly affected by desertification and 1 billion people in more than 100 countries are at risk.

Figure 10: The health impacts of desertification

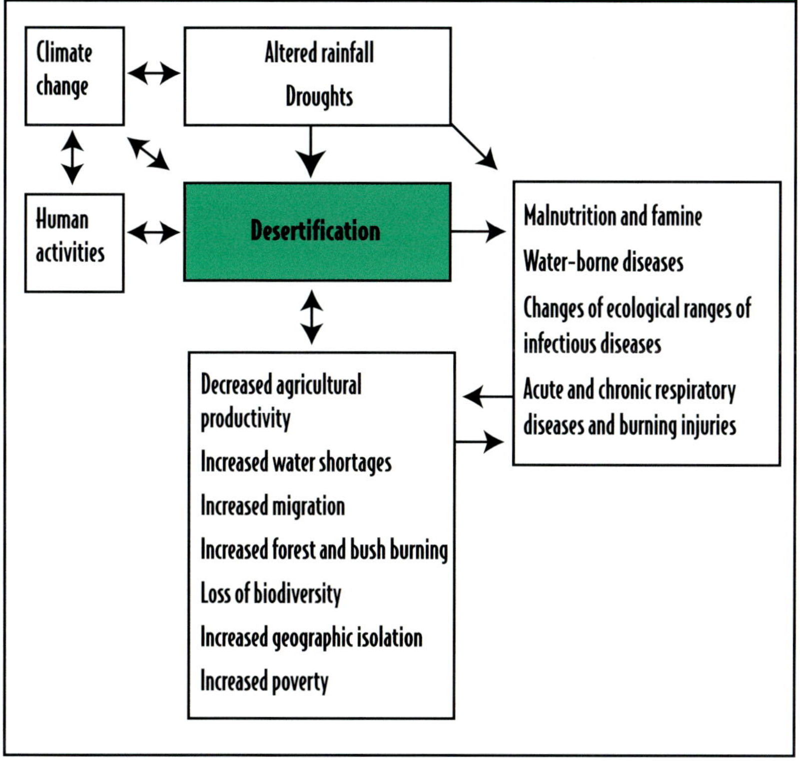

Menne, B. and R. Bertollini, 'The Health Impacts of Desertification and Drought', WHO in United Nations Convention to Combat Desertification in Those Countries Experiencing Serious Drought and/or Desertification, Particularly in Africa (UNCCD), Down to Earth: Newsletter of the UNCCD, No. 14, December 2000.

- Reduction of the land's natural resilience to recover from climatic disturbances;
- Reduction of soil productivity;
- Damaged vegetation cover, such that edible plants can be replaced by non-edible ones;
- Increased downstream flooding, reduced water quality, sedimentation in rivers and lakes and siltation of reservoirs and navigation channels;
- Aggravated health problems due to wind-blown dust, including eye infections, respiratory illnesses, allergies and mental stress;
- Undermined food production; and
- Loss of livelihoods compelling affected people to migrate.

These issues are addressed in the UN Convention to Combat Desertification in Those Countries Experiencing Serious Drought and/or Desertification, Particularly in Africa (UNCCD), which entered into force in December 1996, and to date has been ratified by 179 countries. The Convention is implemented through action programmes, which at the national level address the underlying causes of desertification and drought and identify measures to prevent and reverse it.

Deforestation

More than 110 million hectares of forest, about 11 million hectares a year, disappeared during the 1990s. Most of this loss was in developing countries. About 45 per cent of the world's original forests are gone[10]. Major causes of deforestation and forest degradation lie outside the forest sector and include the need to create agricultural land and to harvest fuel wood for food and energy. Approximately half of the wood harvested in the world is used as fuel wood and charcoal, mostly in developing countries. In developed countries the main uses are for industrial products. The alarming rates of deforestation and the associated loss of environmental resources, social and cultural traditions – alongside the loss of the economic and productive capacity of forestland – account for the fact that forest preservation is now a major priority on the national, regional and global policy and political agendas.

The removal of trees decreases the ability of the soils to absorb and retain water; thus contributing to the depletion of the groundwater aquifers, which supply about one-third of the world's population. Aquifers are the sole source of water for many rural communities worldwide[11]. Cleared lands stripped of their tree cover also are more susceptible to:

- Erosion, which degrades fertile lands and silts waterways, lakes, rivers and coastal waters, thereby degrades water quality for human consumption and disrupts ecosystem processes by choking fish hatcheries, coral reefs, etc.;
- Decreased groundwater recharge because the barren soils do not infiltrate water as effectively;
- Increased malaria transmission, bearing in mind that 90 per cent of the malaria disease burden is linked with underlying environmental factors[12], and claims some 750,000 children under five annually[13]; and
- Desertification and drought (see previous section).

Deforestation is also intrinsically linked to the loss of biodiversity as original rain forests host numerous species of precious fauna and flora (see next section). The significance of protecting rain forests for children cannot be overemphasized. Food security and sustainability of livelihoods as provided by forests are critical to child development. Forests also offer climatic and water resource conservation benefits that directly impact child health. The rich medicinal resources stored in forests are another link to children's welfare.

International efforts in this realm were undertaken through the Intergovernmental Panel on Forests (IPF) and its successor the

Intergovernmental Forum on Forests (IFF). Recently, the international community decided to establish the United Nations Forum on Forests (UNFF), as a new subsidiary body of the United Nations Economic and Social Council (ECOSOC), which is expected to contribute significantly to advancing consensus-building on the many complex issues related to forests.

Loss of Biodiversity

One hundred and fifty years ago, the Native American leader, Chief Seattle, is reported to have said we humans are but a thread in the web of life. He added, whatever we do to the web, "We do to ourselves."

The web is unravelling at an increasing rate. Both plant and animal species have been disappearing at 50 to 100 times the natural rate, due to such factors as the large-scale clearing and burning of forests, over-harvesting of plants and animals, indiscriminate use of pesticides, draining and filling of wetlands, destructive fishing practices, air pollution and the conversion of wild lands to agricultural and urban uses. Recent studies suggest that this high rate of extinction will accelerate even faster, taking an increasing number of living plants and animals away from us forever.

This species loss and ecosystem disruption is causing a complex range of circumstances with consequences to human health. In response, governments and communities worldwide are now concerned with the purification of air and water, maintenance of soil fertility, mitigation of floods and droughts, detoxification and decomposition of wastes, maintaining concentrations of vital gases and water vapour in the atmosphere, and controlling infectious agents in the environment. In addition, the loss of biodiversity obstructs the discovery of new medicines to treat various diseases.

Another emerging modern health concern is biosafety and the effects of advances in and increased use of biotechnology to genetically modify foods. Public concern about the health and ecological risks of foods made with biotechnology has intensified in

Europe and has spread rapidly to other parts of the world, including the United States. Proponents contend that biotechnology could help feed the developing world, cut costs, and reduce the need for pesticides. Detractors say the health risks of the emerging technology are unclear and the environmental hazards potentially alarming. Research is proceeding in order to respond to the many health and environmental questions raised and to guide eventual biotechnology regulations.

The United Nations Convention on Biological Diversity (UNCBD), which was adopted at UNCED in 1992 and has since been ratified by more than 175 countries, establishes three main goals: the conservation of biological diversity, the sustainable use of its components, and the fair and equitable sharing of the benefits from the use of genetic resources. In May 2000, the Convention's Cartagena Protocol on Biosafety was opened for signature. The Protocol seeks to protect the planet's species and ecosystems from the potential risks posed by living modified organisms, commonly referred to as genetically modified organisms, and to establish an advanced informed agreement procedure for ensuring that countries are provided with the information necessary to make informed decisions before agreeing to the import of such organisms. The Protocol has been hailed as a breakthrough from a health and environment perspective in that it is the first global treaty that formally enshrines the "precautionary approach", as set forth in the 1992 Rio Declaration on Environment and Development, as a principle of international environmental law.

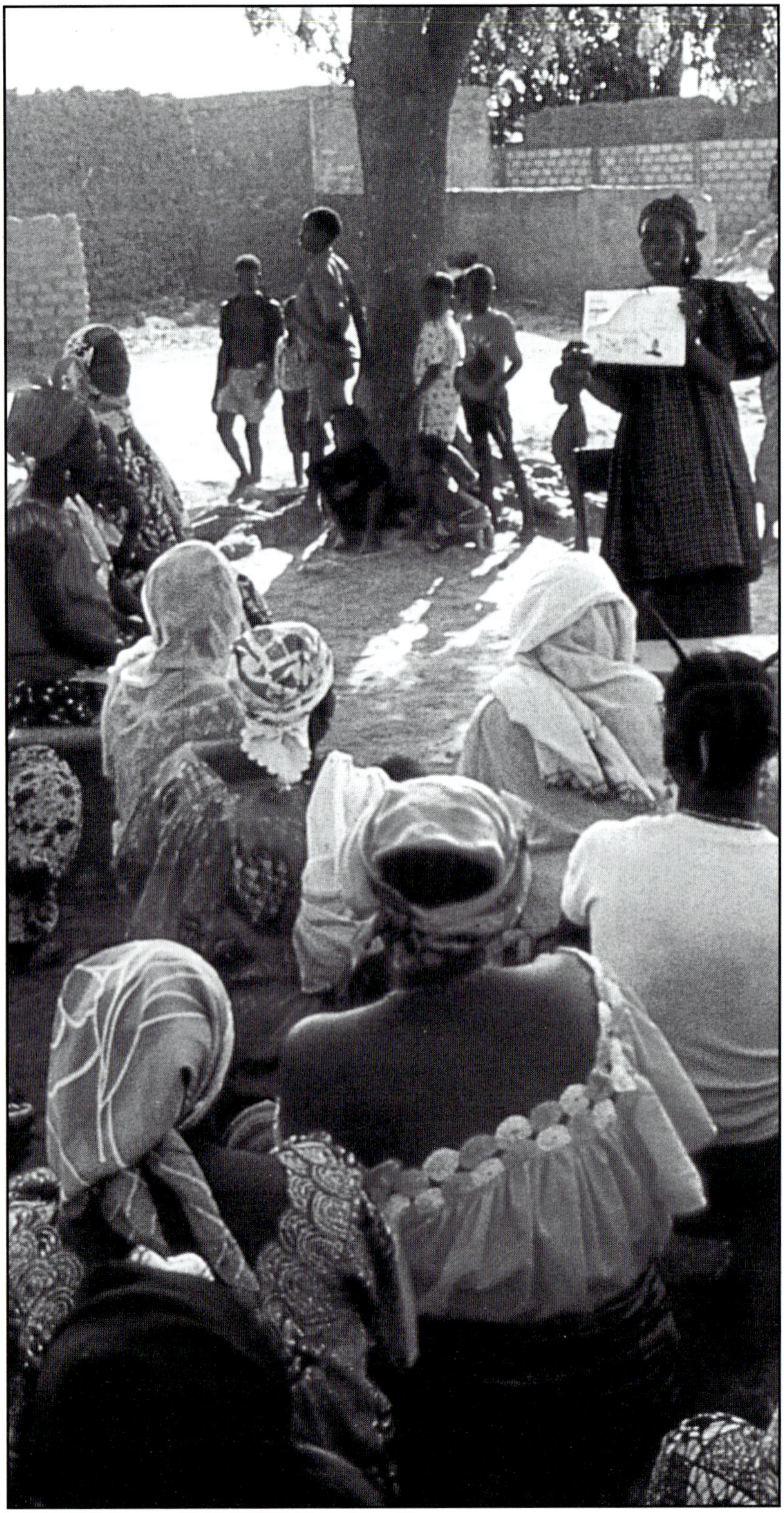

Governments, the United Nations system, civil society and the private sector need to work together to promote safe environments for children.

5 Recommendations

While the linkages between children and the environment have been acknowledged at the international level, including in Agenda 21 and the 1990 Programme of Action of the World Summit for Children (see box 1), sustained progress can only be made if individuals strive together for concerted action. Governments, the United Nations system, civil society and the private sector need to work together to foster intersectoral cooperation at all levels to promote safe environments for children. If at each level of action, policies and strategies are tailored to specific realities and are designed to complement each other, real and cost-effective synergies will be achieved.

To follow up the information offered in the previous chapters with a call to action, this chapter presents a set of broad recommendations to stimulate discussion and intensify action.

Local Initiatives

Community participation and actions at the local and household level are critical because this is where children's health and well-being are first and directly influenced by environmental problems. A safe immediate environment for children depends largely on how well communities and families can manage problems, such as a lack of safe drinking water, unsanitary excreta and refuse disposal, smoky indoor air, crowded living spaces and degraded natural resources.

At this level, environmental health interventions must be very specific, concrete and results-oriented. In addition to the examples of possible local initiatives that were included in chapter 3, below are several suggestions that can be taken by communities and those supporting them in local and national governments, regional partnerships, international organizations and civil society.

At the local level there is a need to:

- Build community capacity (namely, municipalities) to sustainably manage local resources, particularly the essential resources of drinking water and fuel wood. In practical terms, community environmental management aimed at preventing diarrhoeal diseases, malaria and acute respiratory infections (ARIs) – three of the primary child killers – involve actions which inhibit, interrupt, and reduce the generation, transmission, and exposure to disease agents. Examples of possible community- and household-level interventions for reducing incidences of these diseases can be found in table 5.

- Support community-based environmental care in partnership with local NGOs. Activities such as planting trees, vegetable gardening, protecting water sources, building sanitary latrines, recycling and composting domestic wastes, terracing slopes, etc. can both improve local environmental quality and directly benefit children and families.

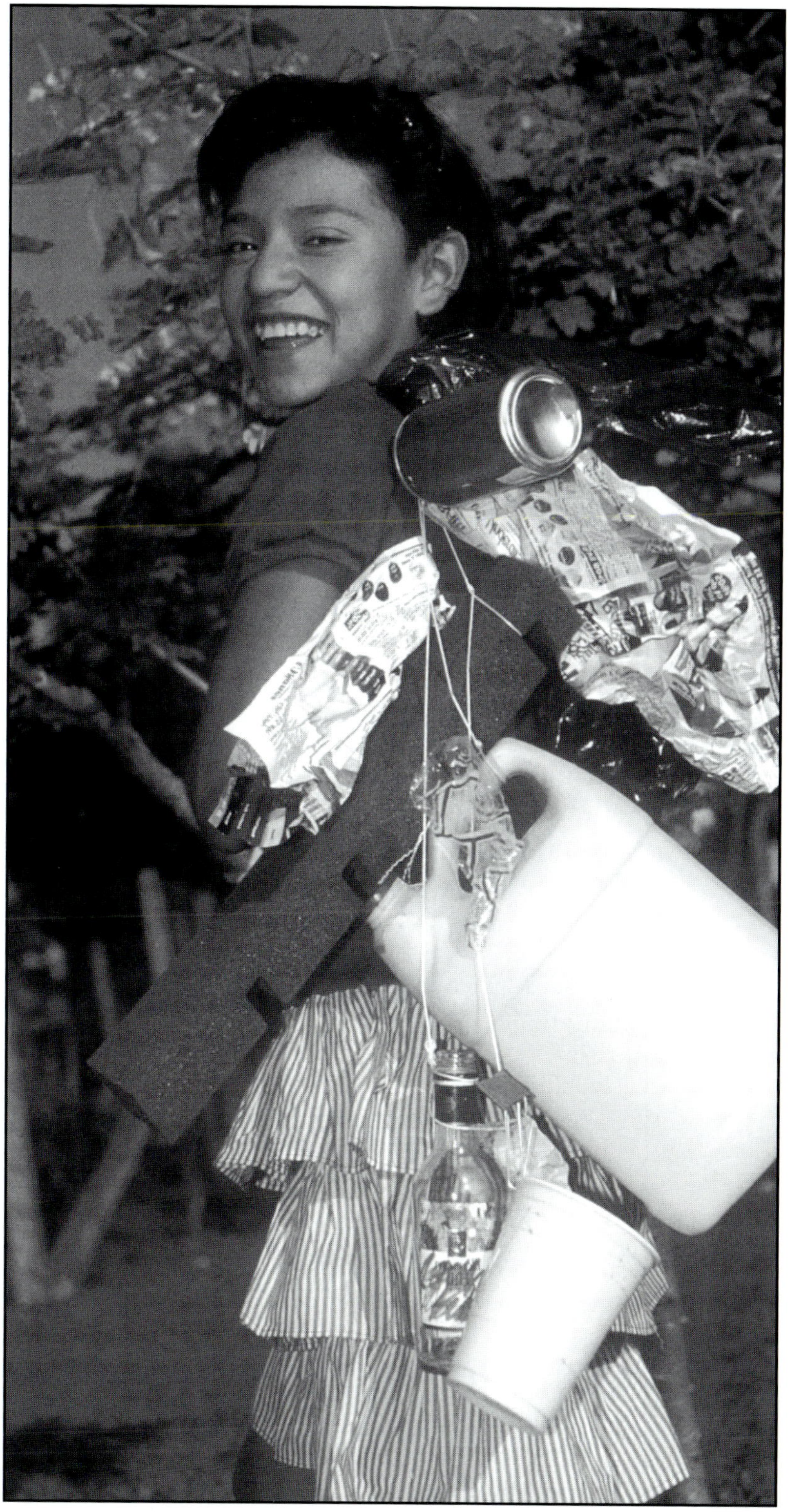

Community participation and actions at the local and household level are critical since this is where children's health and well-being are first and directly influenced by environmental problems.

Table 5: Matrix of Possible Community- and Household-Level Interventions for Reducing Incidences of Diarrhoea, Malaria and ARIs

	Inhibit generation of disease agents	Interrupt transmission of disease agents	Reduce exposure to disease agents
Preventing diarrhoeal disease	■ Proper maintenance of water supplies ■ Protection of food supply ■ Proper food storage ■ Excreta disposal	■ Protection of drinking water ■ Disposal of contaminated food ■ Hand washing ■ Reduction of solid waste ■ Corralling livestock to limit transmission ■ Reduction of fly breeding sites	■ Purification of drinking water ■ Proper cooking time and temperature ■ Proper infant feeding practices ■ Personal protection, e.g. wearing shoes
Preventing malaria	■ Application of larvicide ■ Reduction of breeding sites ■ Appropriate agricultural practices ■ Proper maintenance of water supplies	■ Vector diversion ■ Residual spraying ■ Surveillance/ early treatment to reduce disease reservoir	■ Domestic protection, e.g. screening ■ Personal protection, e.g. bed nets, protective clothes, repellents
Preventing ARIs	■ Use of alternative clean energy and fuels ■ Reduction of burning of solid waste ■ Reduction of agricultural burning	■ Improvement in household ventilation ■ Use of efficient, vented household stoves ■ Street sweeping	■ Reduction of activity on high pollution days ■ Transfer of cooking fires outdoors ■ Keeping children away from smoky stoves

- Promote hygiene awareness and education for a sustainable future using formal and informal channels. Hygiene education can help family members and children establish hygienic behaviour so as to block or at least reduce harmful environmental agents – particularly biological ones – from entering a child's body. Environmental education, if tailored to local situations, will increase mothers' and children's knowledge and ability to protect themselves from environmental hazards. In rural developing areas where literacy rates are usually low, hygiene education and environmental education can be combined and integrated into literacy efforts.
- Increase attention to family-level activities in children's environmental health projects. In most cases, simple and low-cost options exist for parents to take action aimed at lessening environmental risks to their young children.
- Support and build the capacity of parents – both mothers and fathers - in fulfilling their responsibility for providing quality care to their children. Parents should have easy access to up-to-date and correct information on childcare, including children's environmental health issues. There is a need to ensure that adequate care is provided to disadvantaged children in a family, such as a girl child who often experiences gender discrimination or a disabled child.

Note: This chart lists environmental health contributions to an integrated approach to child and maternal health. Other components not mentioned include immunizations, oral rehydration, breastfeeding, safe delivery, birth spacing, micronutrients, and prompt diagnosis and treatment.

Source: Environmental Health Project (sponsored by United States Agency for International Development), "Prevention: Environmental Health Interventions to Sustain Child Survival", Applied Study No. 3. Environmental Health Project, Washington, D.C., 1997.

- Encourage and support children and youth to participate in local environmental management activities, including identifying and monitoring environmental problems and how they relate to livelihoods and taking action to combat specific threats. Environmental education through informal and formal channels can significantly enhance life skills of children. It provides children with environmental knowledge and engenders respect for the world and their role and responsibilities in it (see box 11).

At the national level, the key is to increase understanding of how to mainstream environmental considerations.

National Actions

At the national level, the key is to increase understanding of how to mainstream environmental considerations and to recognize and exploit the interlinkages and synergies between environmental issues and child-focused interventions. There is also a need to fill the substantial gaps that exist in the information and thus the understanding of children's environmental health issues, both through increased and better coordinated research and data collection and through the development and monitoring of indicators to assess progress made in this field.

While many of the recommendations for action at the international and regional levels may also be relevant to national circumstances, certain issues demand specific national level response, for example, to:

- Increase understanding that child health, growth and development depends at least as much on the control of root environmental causes of poor health as on clinical responses to disease. Such understanding should lead to an enhanced preventive aspect in national policies regarding children's health.
- Develop national laws and regulations for the early detection of environmental diseases and increase nations' capacities to implement and uphold them.

Box 11: Top Environmental Trends Among Young People

Young people from all over the world who contributed to Pachamama: Our Earth – Our Future (UNEP, Peace Child International, UNICEF & UNESCO, 1999) were asked to list their top 10 positive trends and top 10 negative ones:

Top 10 Positive Emerging Trends

- Increased recycling
- More reforestation
- Greater animal protection
- More use of solar energy
- Water conservation
- Higher environmental awareness
- More measures against pollution
- More power to NGOs
- More natural food products
- More protection of rainforests

Top 10 Negative Emerging Trends

- Increased pollution
- More deforestation
- Intensified hunting of animals
- More air pollution
- Widening ozone hole
- Worse water pollution
- Water scarcity
- More toxic waste
- Over-population
- Increased amounts of rubbish

Source: United Nations Environment Programme, Peace Child International, United Nations Children's Fund, and United Nations Educational, Scientific and Cultural Organization, Pachamama: Our Earth - Our Future, Evans Brothers Ltd., London, 1997.

- Strengthen intersectoral coordination and cooperation among government departments. Especially, there is a need to reconcile health and environment as prime elements of sustainable development programmes. (See box 12.)

- Put children at the centre of sustainable development agendas. In the context of children's environmental health, this means that national policy and regulation systems need to take into account the special rights and vulnerabilities of children in terms of environmental risk factors. It also means that government spending on child protection, including environmental safety, should be accorded a high priority. Some specific action points may include:

    - Refine current risk assessment methods to better evaluate specific exposure pathways and dose-response characteristics of children when setting protective standards, so as to ensure early detection of diseases;

    - Improve monitoring and assessment of children's health and the environment to expand the knowledge base;

    - Expand national education curricula to include education for a sustainable future, which integrates environmental and hygiene education.

- Develop functional voluntary partnerships between communities, schoolteachers, environmental and public health NGOs, scientific and academic communities, and local and national governments. Partnering with civil society helps to ensure success through sharing of information and follow-up activities.

- Empower and educate health/environment professionals to ensure a better recognition of environmental health problems affecting children. Incorporate children's environmental health issues into the teaching curricula of medical and clinical toxicology university courses.

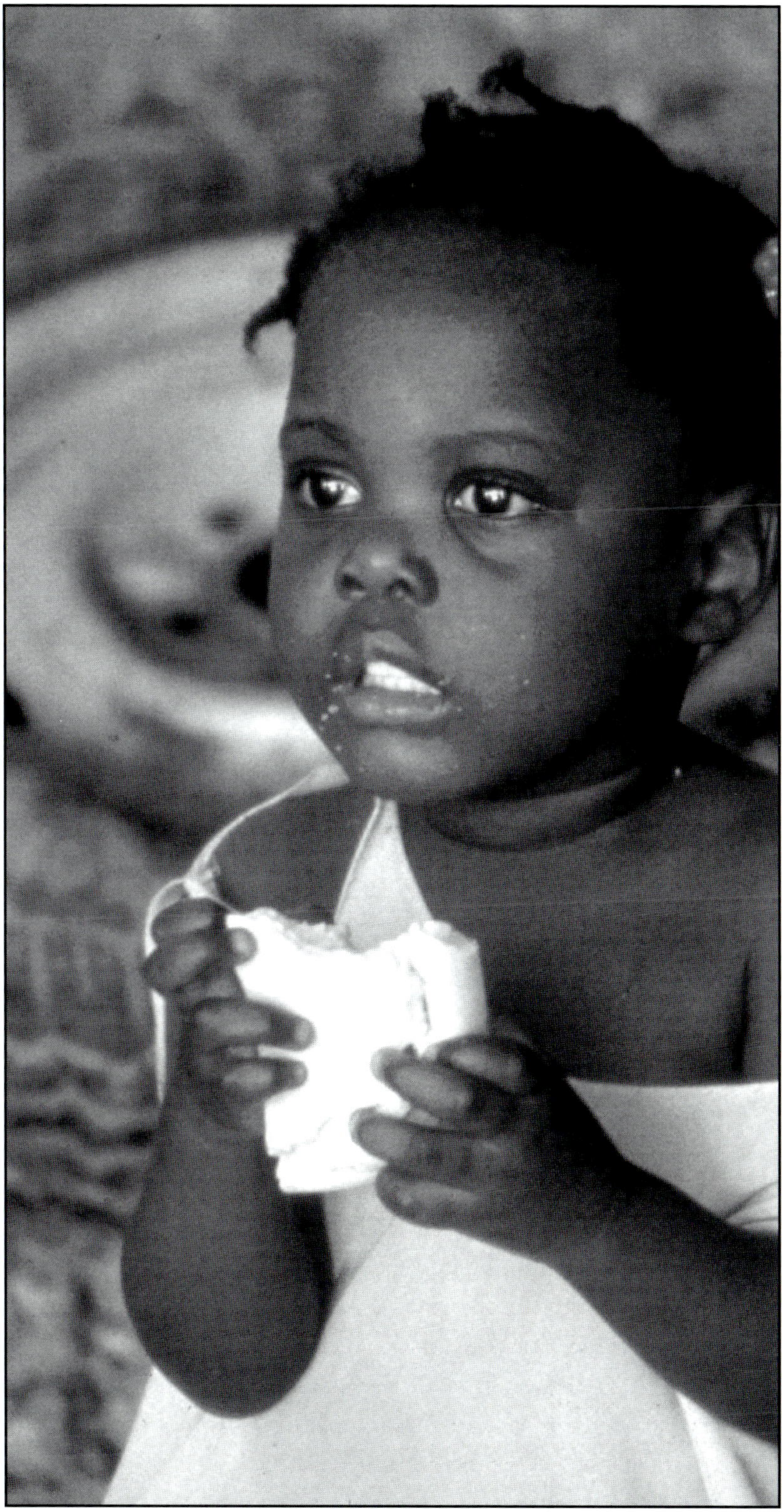

Government spending on child protection, including environmental safety, should be accorded a high priority.

- Give special policy attention to disadvantaged children, who are generally closer and more vulnerable to environmental hazards. These children may include girls, working children, homeless children, orphans, disabled children, children displaced by armed conflicts, children living in extreme poverty, children of urban slums, children affected by HIV/AIDS, and children caught in violence, sexual abuse or drug use.

Regional Partnerships

Countries can benefit substantially from regional consultations and collaboration where they can exchange ideas and best practices.

Most of the recommendations put forth in the next section for the international level also apply at the regional level. There are, however, two points that retain specific regional relevance, which are highlighted below. At the regional level there is a need to:

- Develop coordinated regional approaches to children's environmental health issues. Nations in a particular region often face similar environmental threats and many are both multi-causal and transboundary in nature. Likewise, children from countries within a region often face similar social and economic situations. Therefore, countries can benefit substantially from regional consultations and collaboration where they can exchange ideas and best practices and replicate measures to effectively mitigate environmental threats to the health of their populations. Regional consultations are also vital to fashion policy responses to specific environmental threats that are plaguing a particular area beyond any one national border (see box 13).
- Pay special attention to regional priority environmental problems that most afflict children of the region. Children of different regions often face unique environmental threats, which should not be neglected while dealing with high-profile global issues. The lack of safe drinking water and basic sanitation facilities, for instance, is perhaps the most dismal environmental condition endured by the majority of Asian and African children.

Box 12: An Initiative to Protect Children's Environmental Health

In 1997, the United States Environmental Protection Agency established the Office of Children's Health Protection (OCHP) to implement their commitment to protect children from environmental health hazards. OCHP's mission is to make the protection of children's health a fundamental goal of public health and environmental protection in the United States. This is enabling multi-agency cooperation within the federal government and in collaboration with the NGO community and has resulted in varied efforts, such as:

- The Food and Quality Protection Act, passed unanimously by Congress to protect children from microbial contamination;
- The Asthma Strategy, a multiple agency effort to address asthma and the environment;
- The Lead Strategy, also a multiple agency effort to address the problem of children with higher than advisable blood lead levels;
- Outreach and education efforts;
- Research centres and the research agenda devoted to children's environmental health issues; and
- Paediatric environmental health specialty units

Source: The United States Environmental Protection Agency: http://www.epa.gov/children

Box 13: Examples of Regional Efforts

- In 1999 a major ministerial conference was held on environment and health in Europe under the auspices of WHO, which produced the London Declaration on Action in Partnership. It marked a new commitment to action in partnership for improving the environment and health in the 21st century. The ministers and representatives of the European Member States committed "to develop policies and implement actions to provide children with a safe environment, including during prenatal and postnatal development, towards the highest attainable level of health."
- In June 2000, the North American Commission on Environmental Cooperation Council (comprised of the top environmental officials from Canada, Mexico and USA) passed a council resolution on children's health and the environment. The resolution commits the Parties to develop a cooperative agenda to protect children from environmental threats, and, among other activities, calls for the formation of an Expert Advisory Board to provide advice to the council on these matters.
- In 2001 in Kuala Lumpur, South-East Asian nations met to negotiate an agreement designed to prevent a repeat of the forest fires and their devastating haze that beset the region in 1997 and 1998 and caused significant health problems. Regionally integrated approaches such as these, engineered around the concept of prevention, can significantly help to reduce environmental health threats to children.
- In collaboration with several governmental and international organizations, WHO organized an international conference entitled Environmental Threats to the Health of Children: Hazards and Vulnerability held in Bangkok, Thailand in March 2002. The scope

of the conference was largely regional and focused on Children's Environmental Health (CEH) issues that had the highest prevalence and health impact in South East Asia and Western Pacific Regions. It presented and discussed recent knowledge and new research results and methodologies used to identify the effects of environmental threats to children's health. The purpose was to increase health and environment professionals' awareness of the effects of pollution on children's health and development and to motivate the required action. The major outcomes of the conference included a statement setting priorities for action and a commitment to national and international activities in the area of CEH.

International Support

In the past decade, several international agreements (see box 1) have recognized the link between children's well-being and the protection of the environment. Despite this, there is a need to bring children's environmental health, growth, and development issues to the forefront of the international agenda and translate these declarations into concrete action (see box 14). At the international level there is a need to, among other things:

- Ensure that children's rights as well as their special vulnerabilities are systematically taken into account in discussions and negotiations on environmental issues. Such recognition needs to generate more specific policy decisions and actions directed to children's particular needs.
- Fully recognize the important role of environmental protection in child survival, development and protection. Global efforts for children need to adopt the concept of protecting the child's environment and to strengthen and

integrate into their child-related programmes appropriate environmental interventions that will improve a child's immediate environment.

- Further develop international environmental law that will safeguard children's health, growth and development from environmental risk factors. The existing and rapidly expanding body of international environmental conventions and protocols play a key role in addressing the most pressing global environmental challenges, which threaten human health including that of children. Commitments need to be honoured and implementation needs to be accelerated.
- Employ a precautionary approach in dealing with environmental issues, as this will widely be in the best interest of children and future generations. A lack of full scientific certainty should not be used as a reason for postponing cost-effective measures to prevent environmental degradation.
- Develop and build consensus on children's environmental health indicators. Just as basic economic indicators have been instrumental to Governments in estimating and steering the functioning of national and world economies, we need effective and user-friendly indicators to monitor and protect children from environmental health threats. Actions to protect children from environmental hazards will be, at the best, arbitrary and unsystematic until a core set of good indicators can be widely adopted. Since indicators receive media attention, they can also play a crucial role in bringing the public's focus to the issue. Most importantly, such indicators will provide a sound basis for children's environmental health policies.
- Encourage and promote national investment in early childhood care, including the improvement of home, school and community environments. The quality of the environment exerts a powerful influence on whether a child will survive his or her first years. Therefore, improv-

ing the local environmental conditions can be effective in reducing childhood malnutrition and disease and can ultimately break the inter-generational transmission of poverty.

- Raise awareness of various stakeholders and children's environmental health, growth and development issues. This will involve efforts to:
  - Disseminate concise information to decision-makers and all those caring for children, which can help to stimulate feasible actions at all levels to reduce child exposure to environmental pollutants.
  - Promote, support and coordinate research, monitoring and assessment with regard to children's special vulnerabilities to environmental degradation, in order to yield the required information for effective decision-making (at each level of competence). The knowledge gaps related to children's environmental health are substantial.
  - Coordinate existing efforts and initiatives that specifically address children's environmental health issues, creating coherent networks for action. Establish active partnerships among the various stakeholder groups: Governments, civil society (i.e.: non-governmental organizations, foundations, private institutions, community groups, universities, research centres, etc.) media and international organizations.

Box 14: Examples of International Efforts

- In 1997, UNICEF and UNEP signed a Memorandum of Understanding that facilitates cooperation primarily in terms of advocacy in areas of common concern and in scientific/technical cooperation on programme activities. The MOU also commits the two organizations to support programme implementation through the best scientific and environmental information that bears on children and child health, especially at the field level in developing countries.
- In 1999, WHO set up a Task Force for the Protection of Children's Environmental Health. The objectives are to prevent disease and disability associated with chemical and physical threats to children, taking into consideration biological risks in the environment and acknowledging the importance of social and psychosocial factors. To achieve this, the Task Force promotes activities on the identification, assessment, mitigation and prevention of, as well as communication about, environmental threats.
- In 1999, WHO and UNEP signed a Memorandum of Understanding with a view to strengthening their cooperation in the field of environmental health as an essential factor in achieving sustainable development.
- UNICEF has been supporting an international initiative on School Sanitation and Hygiene Education (SSHE) within an inter-agency effort called the FRESH framework (Focusing Resources on Effective School Health). The World Bank, UNICEF, WHO and UNESCO are among the active members of FRESH. SSHE focuses on using a life-skills approach to hygiene education, improving the sanitary and environmental conditions of schools, and providing outreach to families and communities. Improved hygiene and sanitation in schools help encourage girls to attend schools and improve the health of pupils and their ability to learn. UNICEF-supported

SSHE activities are taking place in over 40 countries across Africa, Asia, Latin America and the Caribbean.

- In September 2001, two NGOs, the Canadian Institute of Child Health and the U.S. Children's Environmental Health Network, hosted their second 'Global Forum' on children's environmental health in Washington D.C. The Global Forum focused on the special vulnerability of children and how the environment in which they live, learn, work and play impacts them. It attracted public health specialists, medical practitioners, scientific researchers, government officials, policy makers, industry, advocacy groups and community-based organizations.

Multilateral Environmental Agreements (MEAs)

At the international level, the rapidly expanding body of international environmental law is a key component in the international community's reservoir of policy responses to environment and health threats. MEAs can help to promote innovative policy responses and to enhance processes to address the most pressing environmental challenges that threaten human health. To date, it is estimated that there are more than 500 international treaties and agreements related to the environment. The existence of such legally binding agreements is a remarkable feat of the global community, clearly indicating a collective will and commitment to protecting the environment and, by extension, children's health. A recent example: Governments recognized that persistent organic pollutants (POPs) endanger human health globally as well as the environment from one generation to the next. Hence, they negotiated and signed the Stockholm Convention on POPs to minimize and eliminate some of the most toxic chemicals ever created in order to secure the health of future generations and the integrity of the chain of life.

While current understanding of the linkages between children and the environment has advanced considerably, we must recognize that so much more still needs to be achieved.

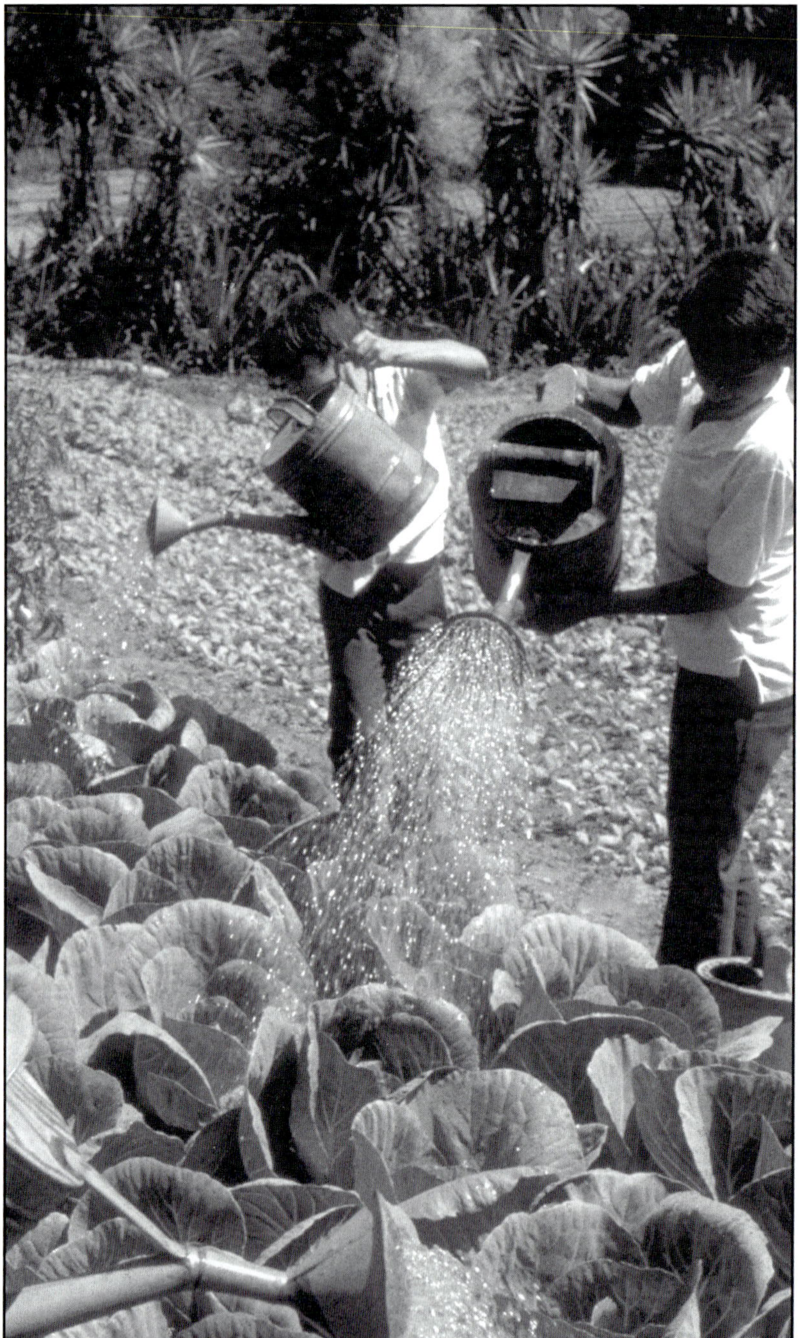

6 Looking Ahead

Ten years have passed since UNEP and UNICEF published the first report on 'Children and the Environment'. At the dawn of the new millennium, while current understanding of the linkages between children and the environment has advanced considerably, we must recognize that so much more still needs to be achieved. For the most part, we know what to do: protect children from environmental health threats and protect the environment to safeguard children's health and their future. In order for this wishful thinking to become reality, consideration for the environment must increasingly be integrated into the strategies addressing childhood development at the international, regional, national, and local levels – and likewise, children's rights and their special vulnerabilities must be fully recognized within environmental management endeavours.

Between two intergovernmental events addressing related aspects of the sustainable development agenda – the Special Session of the United Nations General Assembly on Children in May 2002 and the World Summit on Sustainable Development in

August 2002 – unique opportunities exist to strengthen the interlinkages between children's health and the sustainable management of the environment. This can be done while fighting poverty through efforts to achieve sustainable development.

The goals set for the world's children and sustainable development are within reach, if today's leaders can step up efforts to mobilize collective will, resources, and the wisdom to act early and decisively in the name of children and for future generations. We owe it to our children to ensure a brighter and safer future in this new millennium.

Endnotes

Chapter 1: The Context

[1] United Nations Children's Fund, *The State of the World's Children 2002,* table 1, UNICEF, New York, 2002.

[2] Satterthwaite, David et al., *The Environment for Children,* United Nations Children's Fund and Earthscan Publication, New York, 1996.

[3] United Nations Children's Fund, *First Call for Children: World Declaration and Plan of Action from the World Summit for Children* and *The Convention on the Rights of the Child,* UNICEF, New York, 1990.

[4] United Nations Children's Fund, *Progress since the World Summit for Children: A Statistical Review,* page 2, UNICEF, New York, September 2001.

[5] Ibid. page 26.

[6] Ibid. page 5.

[7] Ibid. page 10.

[8] Grant, James P. (Executive Director of UNICEF), Address to the United Nations Conference on Environment and Development, United Nations Children's Fund, New York, 1992.

[9] World Meteorological Organization and others, *Comprehensive Assessment of the Freshwater Resources of the World*, WMO, cited in UNEP, Global Environment Outlook 2000, Earthscan Publication, London, 1999.

[10] United Nations Secretariat of the Convention to Combat Desertification: http://www.unccd.int/main.php

[11] United Nations Environment Programme, *Global Ministerial Environment Forum, Policy Issues: Emerging Policy Issues*, Discussion paper presented by the Executive Director, UNEP/GC.21/5,18 January 2001.

[12] World Health Organization, *Health and Environment in Sustainable Development: Five Years after the Earth Summit*, WHO, Geneva, 1997.

[13] World Health Organization, World Health Report 1999 Database: http://www.who.int/violence_injury_prevention/injury/InjuryBofDtables.htm World and United Nations Children's Fund, Sanitation for All: Promoting Dignity and Human Rights, UNICEF, New York, 2000.

[14] United Nations, *Report of the Secretary General on We the Children: End-Decade Review of Follow-up to the World Summit for Children*, New York, 2001.

[15] Ibid.

[16] United Nations Centre for Human Settlements (Habitat), *Cities in a Globalizing World – Global Report on Human Settlements 2001*, Earthscan Publications, London, 2001.

[17] Ibid.

[18] United Nations Centre for Human Settlements (Habitat), *The State of the World's Cities 2001*, UNCHS (Habitat), 2001.

[19] Ibid.

[20] United Nations Environment Programme, *Global Ministerial Environment Forum, Policy Issues: Emerging Policy Issues*, op. cit.

Chapter 2: A Child's World and Life Cycle

[1] World Health Organization, World Health Report 1999 Database, op. cit.

[2] Commission on the Nutrition Challenges of the 21st Century, *Ending Malnutrition by 2020: An agenda for change in the millennium*, final report to the ACC/SCN, cited in UNICEF, *The State of the World's Children 2001*, UNICEF, New York, 2001.

[3] World Supply and Sanitation Collaborative Council, *Global Environmental Sanitation Initiative: Sanitation for All*, an advocacy brochure, WSSC, 2000.

[4] World Health Organization, World Health Report 1999 Database, op. cit.

[5] Faustman, Elaine M. et al., "Mechanisms Underlying Children's Susceptibility to Environmental Toxicants", *Environmental Health Perspectives*, Vol.108, Suppl.1, 2000.

[6] Ibid.

[7] United Nations Children's Fund and United Nations Environment Programme, *Childhood Lead Poisoning: Information for Advocacy and Action*, UNICEF and UNEP, New York, 1997.

[8] Schroeder, Stephen R., "Mental Retardation and Developmental Disabilities Influenced by Environmental Neurotoxic Insults", *Environmental Health Perspectives*, Vol. 108, Supplement 3, 2000.

[9] Mott, Lawrie et al., *Our Children at Risk: The 5 worst environmental threats to their health*, Natural Resource Defense Council, New York, 1997.

[10] Ibid.

[11] United Nations Environment Programme, United Nations Children's Fund, World Health Organization and Food and Agriculture Organization, *Childhood Pesticide Poisoning: Information for Advocacy and Action* (draft), UNEP, UNICEF, WHO & FOA, New York, 2001.

[12] Weiss, Bernard, "Vulnerability of Children and the Developing Brain to Neurotoxic Hazards.", *Environmental Health Perspectives*, Vol. 108, Supplement 3, 2000.

[13] Bloom, B.S., *Stability and Change in Human Characteristics*, John Wiley & Sons, New York, 1964.

[14] Carnegie Task Force on Meeting the Needs of Young Children., *Starting Points: Meeting the Needs of Our Youngest Children*, Carnegie Corporation of New York, New York, 1994.

[15] Young, Mary Eming, *Early Child Development: Investing in the Future*, The World Bank, Washington, D.C., 1996.

[16] United Nations Children's Fund, *Sanitation for All: Promoting Dignity and Human Rights*, UNICEF, New York, 2000.

[17] World Health Organization, World Health Report 1999 Database, op.cit.

[18] Children's Environmental Health Network (CEHN): http://www.cehn.org

[19] Ibid.

[20] United States Environmental Protection Agency, *The EPA Children's Environmental Health Yearbook Supplement*, EPA, Washington, D.C., 2000.

[21] Zahm, S.H. and S. S. Devesa, "Childhood Cancer: Overview of Incidence Trends and Environmental Carcinogens.", *Environmental Health Perspectives*, Vol.103, Suppl.6, pp.177-184, 1995; Weinstein, I.B., "The Origins of Human Cancer: Molecular Mechanism of Carcinogenesis and Their Treatment," *Cancer Research*, Vol.48, pp.4135-4143, 1988; National Research Council, *Pesticides in the Diets of Infants and Children*, NRC, National Academy Press, Washington, D.C., 1993.

[22] United Nations Children's Fund, *The State of the World's Children 2001*, UNICEF, New York, 2001.

[23] Lonergan, Steve, "The Role of Environmental Degradation in Population Displacement", *Environmental Change and Security Project Report*, Iss.4, pp.5-15, 1998. http://ecsp.si.edu/pdf/Report4b.pdf

[24] United Nations, *Report of the Secretary General on We the Children: End-Decade Review of Follow-up to the World Summit for Children*, op. cit.

Chapter 3: Environmental Threats to Children

[1] World Health Organization, United Nations Children's Fund, Water Supply and Sanitation Collaborative Council, *Global Water Supply and Sanitation Assessment 2000*, op. cit.

[2] United Nations Environment Programme, *Global Environment Outlook 2000*, Earthscan Publications, London, 1999. op. cit.

[3] Ibid.

[4] Ibid.

[5] Ibid.

[6] Ibid.

[7] World Health Organization, United Nations Children's Fund, Water Supply and Sanitation Collaborative Council, *Global Water Supply and Sanitation Assessment 2000*, op. cit.

[8] Vrijheid, Martine, "Health Effects of Residence Near Hazardous Waste Landfill Sites: A Review of Epidemiologic Literature", *Environmental Health Perspectives*, Vol. 108, Suppl.1, 2000.

[9] Vrijheid, Martine, H. Dolk, B. Armstrong et al., "Chromosomal congenital anomalies and residence near hazardous waste landfill sites", *The Lancet*, Vol. 359, pp. 320-22, 2002. The researchers studied 245 cases of children born with chromosomal defects and 2,412 healthy babies who lived near 23 landfill sites in five European countries. They concluded that people living within 1.8 miles (0-3 km) of a landfill had a higher chance of having a child with a chromosomal defect than couples living further away. However, more study is needed to fully understand the exact role of chemical pollutants.

[10] World Health Organization, United Nations Children's Fund, Water Supply and Sanitation Assessment, *Global Water Supply and Sanitation Assessment 2000*, op. cit.

[11] World Health Organization, United Nations Children's Fund, Water Supply and Sanitation Assessment, *Global Water Supply and Sanitation Assessment 2000*, op. cit.

[12] Ibid.

[13] Ibid.

[14] United Nations Children's Fund, *Sanitation for All: Promoting Dignity and Human Rights*, op. cit.

[15] World Health Organization, *World Health Report 1999* Database, op. cit.

[16] Ibid.

[17] United Nations Children's Fund, *Rolling Back Malaria*, UNICEF, New York, 1999.

[18] Economic and Social Council of the United Nations, *Health and Sustainable Development: Report of the Secretary General to the Commission on Sustainable Development, Economic and Social Council*, E/CN.17/2001, New York, 2001.

[19] Gubler, Duane J., "Resurgent Vector-Borne Diseases as a Global Health Problem", *Emerging Infectious Diseases*, Vol.4, No.3, 1998.

[20] World Health Organization, *Health and Environment in Sustainable Development: Five Years after the Earth Summit*, table 5.14, WHO, Geneva, 1997.

[21] United Nations Children's Fund, presentation of Kul C. Gautam to the Second Substantive Session of the Preparatory Committee of the Special Session of the United Nations General Assembly on Children, UNICEF, New York, 2001.

[22] Environmental Health Project (sponsored by United States Agency for International Development), *Preventing Child Diarrhoeal Disease – Options for Action*, Washington, D.C, 1999.

[23] Economic and Social Council of the United Nations, *Health and Sustainable Development: Report of the Secretary General to the Commission on Sustainable Development*, op. cit.

[24] World Resources Institute, United Nations Environment Programme, United Nations Development Programme, World Bank, *World Resources 1998-1999 A Guide to the Global Environment: Environmental Change and Human Health*, Oxford University Press, New York, 1998.

[25] Trichiasis, an eye condition caused by chronic inflammation of the inner eyelid, characterised by shrinking eyelid, inward turning of eye-lashes, and cornea scraping.

[26] Wolfson, Elaine M. and Lori Fedewa, Stacie A. Young, *Trachoma: A Women's Health Issue*, (revised), Global Alliance for Women's Health, New York, 1999.

[27] World Health Organization, *Strengthening Interventions to Reduce Helminth Infections: As an Entry Point for the Development of Health-Promoting Schools*, WHO Information Series on School Health, Doc.1, Geneva, 1997.

[28] World Health Organization, *Water for Health: Taking Charge*, WHO, Geneva, 2001.

[29] Ibid.

[30] United Nations Children's Fund, *Rolling Back Malaria*, op. cit.

[31] World Health Organization, *World Health Report 1999 Database*, op. cit.

[32] Wargo, John, *Our Children's Toxic Legacy*, Yale University Press, New Haven, cited in World Resources Institute, United Nations Environment Programme, United Nations Development Programme, and World Bank, *World Resources 1998-1999 A Guide to the Global Environment: Environmental Change and Human Health*, 1998.

[33] United Nation's Children's Fund, *Rolling Back Malaria*, op. cit.

[34] Okenu, Daniel M.N., "An Integrated Approach for Malaria Control in Africa", *Malaria and Infectious Disease in Africa*, 10: 4-13, 1999. http://www.malaria.org/OkenuMalariaControl.html

[35] Kit, Lam Sai, "Japanese encephalitis," Malaysian Medical Association Newsletter, Vol.29, No.1, January, 1999.
http://www.geocities.com/HotSprings/2188/jelsk.html

[36] Gubler, Duane J., "Resurgent Vector-Borne Diseases as a Global Health Problem," Emerging Infectious Diseases, Vol. 4, No.3, 1998.

[37] World Health Organization, Water for Health: Taking Charge, op. cit.

[38] Esrey, S.A. et al., "Effects of improved water supply and sanitation on ascaris, diarrhoea, dracunculiasis, hookworm infection, schistosomiasis, and trachoma", Bulletin of the World Health Organization, 69(5):609-621, 1991.

[39] World Health Organization, *Water for Health: Taking Charge*, op. cit.

[40] United States Environmental Protection Agency: http://www.epa.gov/safewater/kids/child.html

[41] World Health Organization, *Water for Health: Taking Charge*, op. cit.

[42] Ibid.

[43] United Nations Environment Programme, *Global Ministerial Environment Forum, Policy Issues: Emerging Policy Issues*, op. cit.

[44] World Resources Institute, United Nations Environment Programme, United Nations Develop Programme, World Bank, *World Resources 1998-1999 A Guide to the Global Environment: Environmental Change and Human Health*, op. cit.

[45] Ibid.

[46] Satterthwaite et al, *The Environment for Children*, op. cit.

[47] United Nations Children's Fund and United Nations Environment Programme, *Childhood Lead Poisoning: Information for Advocacy and Action*, op. cit.

[48] Walsh, Michael, "The Global Phaseout of Leaded Gasoline: A Successful Initiative," Earth Summit Watch, 1999. http://www.earth-summitwatch.org/gasoline.html.

[49] Ibid.

[50] Myers, Gary J. and Philip W. Davidson, "Does Methylmercury Have a Role in Causing Developmental Disabilities in Children?", *Environmental Health Perspectives*, Vol.108, Suppl.3, 2000.

[51] United State Environmental Protection Agency, Press Release: www.epa.gov/mercury/fish.htm

[52] Myers, Gary J. and Philip W. Davidson, "Does Methylmecury Have a Role in Causing Disabilities in Children?" *Environment Health Perspectives*, op. cit.

[53] Ibid.

[54] United Nations Environment Programme, *Global Environment Outlook 2000*, op. cit.

[55] Ibid.

[56] Food and Agriculture Organization, FAOSTAT Statistics Database, FAO, Rome, Italy, 1997. www.fao.org

[57] United Nations Environment Programme, *Global Environment Outlook 2000*, op. cit.

[58] The information used in this paragraph is from several common sources, such as the US EPA Web site and medical handbooks.

[59] United Nations Children's Fund, *Arsenic Mitigation in Bangladesh* – Media Brief, UNICEF Bangladesh, Dhaka, 2000.

[60] Ibid.

[61] World Health Organization, *World Water Day 2001*: http://www.worldwaterday.org/thematic/natural.html#fluoride

[62] United Nations Children's Fund: http://www.unicef.org/programme/wes/info

[63] Ibid.

[64] World Health Organization, *Report of the World Health Organization: Depleted Uranium Mission to Kosovo*, 2001. http://www.who.int/peh/Radiation

[65] World Health Organization: http://www.who.int/peh/Radiation/radindex.htm (updated on June 8, 2001)

[66] World Health Organization, *Health Consequences of the Chernobyl Accident: Results of the IPHECA Pilot Projects and Related National Programmes*, 1995.

[67] Ibid.

[68] World Health Organization, *Electromagnetic Fields and Public Health, Fact Sheet N183* (revised), 1998.

[69] Ibid.

[70] Ibid.

[71] World Health Organization, *Health and Environment in Sustainable Development: Five Years after the Earth Summit*, op. cit.

[72] Human Rights Watch, *Underage and Unprotected: Child Labor in Egypt's Cotton Fields*, Vol.13, No.1 (E), New York, January 2001.

[73] Walsh, Michael, "The Global Phaseout of Leaded Gasoline: A Successful Initiative", *Earth Summit Watch*, op. cit.

[74] Bates, N. and N. Edwards, J. Roper, G. Volans, *Paediatric Toxicology: Handbook of Poisoning in Children*, Macmillan Reference Ltd, London, 1997.

[75] Carpenter et al., "Environmental Threats to Children: The Asian Perspective," *Environmental Health Perspectives*, Vol.108, No.10, 2000.

[76] World Health Organization, *Health and Environment in Sustainable Development: Five Years after the Earth Summit*, op. cit.

[77] Inter-Organization Programme for the Sound Management of Chemicals, United Nations Environment Programme, United Nations Children's Fund, United Nations Institute for Training and Research, *Global Opportunities for Reducing the Use of Leaded Gasoline*, UNEP Chemicals, Switzerland, 1998.

[78] United States Environmental Protection Agency, *Lead Phase-Out*, 5 July 2000. www.epa.gov/oia/tips/lead2.htm

[79] Reuters/Planet Ark,20 April 2001.

[80] United Nations (Department for Economic and Social Affairs), "Eliminating Mercury Pollution", *Sustainable Development Success Stories*, 1998. http://www.un.org/esa/sustdev/success/mer_pol.htm

[81] United Nations Environment Programme, *Global Ministerial Environment Forum, Policy Issues: Emerging Policy Issues*, op. cit.

[82] World Health Organization, *Health and Environment in Sustainable Development: Five Years after the Earth Summit*, op. cit.

[83] von Schirnding, Yasmin and Nigel Bruce, "Household Energy Use, Health and Development," Background Paper prepared for the USAID/WHO Global Consultation on Indoor Air Pollution and Household Energy in Developing Countries, Washington D. C., 2000.

[84] Hall and Rosillo-Calle, "Biomass in Developing Countries," report to the Office of Technology Assessment, Washington D.C, 1991.

[85] GTZ, "Household energy program 1997" cited in von Schirnding and Bruce, op. cit.

[86] For example, United States Environmental Protection Agency's standards recommend that in only 1% of 24-hour periods should ambient levels of PM10 (small particles of diameter less than 10 microns) exceed 150 mg/m3.

[87] Bruce, Nigel, "Lowering Exposure of Children to Indoor Air Pollution to Prevent ARI: The Need for Information and Action," *Environmental Health Project (EHP) Capsule Report*, No.3, 1999; Smith, K.R. and Youcheng Liu, "Indoor Air Pollution in Developing Countries," Jonathan M. ed., *The Epidemiology of Lung Cancer*, Marcel Dekker Publishing, New York, 1992.

[88] Holdren, John P. and Kirk R. Smith, "Energy, the Environment and Health," *Energy and the Challenge of Sustainability*, United Nations Development Programme, New York, 2000.

[89] Garenne, M., C. Ronsmans, and H. Campbell, "The Magnitude of Mortality from Acute Respiratory Infections in Children under 5 Years in Developing Countries", *World Health Statistics Quarterly*, 45:180-191, 1992 cited in WHO, *Health and Environment in Sustainable Development: Five Years after the Earth Summit*, op. cit.

[90] World Health Organization, *Health and Environment in Sustainable Development*, op. cit.

[91] Holdren, John P. and Kirk R. Smith, "Energy, the Environment and Health," *Energy and the Challenge of Sustainability*, op. cit.

[92] World Health Organization, *Health and Environment in Sustainable Development*, op. cit.

[93] World Health Organization, *World Health Report 1999 Data Base*, op. cit.

[94] Smith, K.R. and Sumi Mehta, "The Burden of Disease from Indoor Air Pollution in Developing Countries: Comparison of Estimates" paper presented at the *Global Consultation: The Health Impact of Indoor Air Pollution and Household Energy in Developing Countries: Setting the Agenda for Action, Summary Report for Participants*, sponsored by USAID and WHO, Washington, D. C., 2000.

[95] Holdren, John, P. and Kirk R. Smith, "Energy, the Environment and Health," *Energy and the Challenge of Sustainability*, op. cit.

[96] *Environmental Health Perspectives*, Vol.106, No.1, January 1998.

[97] Neufeld, Ellis J., A study published in 2 Sept. 1997 issue of Circulation, cited in *Environmental Health Perspectives*, Vol.106, No.1 January 1998.

[98] McConnell, Rob, Kiros Berhane et al., "Asthma in exercising children exposed to ozone: a cohort study", *The Lancet*; Vol. 359: 386-91, 2002.

[99] World Health Organization, *World Health Report 1999 Database*, op. cit.

[100] United Nations Environment Programme, *Global Ministerial Environment Forum, Policy Issues: Emerging Policy Issues*, op. cit.

[101] Agence France-Presse, October 30, 2001.

[102] The United States Environmental Protection Agency: http://www.epa.gov/children/asthma.htm

[103] Levine, J.S., T. Bobbe et al., *Wildland Fires and the Environment: A Global Synthesis,* United Nations Environment Programme, UNEP/DEIAEW/TR.99-1, Nairobi, 1999.

[104] World Bank Press Release, 18 April 2001.

[105] Alliance to End Childhood Lead Poisoning and the Environmental Defense Fund, *The Global Dimensions of Lead Poisoning,* op. cit.

[106] Misana, Salome, "Lessons from the field", *Generating Opportunities: Case Studies on Energy and Women,* pp 17-26, United Nations Development Programme, New York, 2001.

[107] Holdren, John P. and Kirk R. Smith, "Energy, the Environment and Health," *Energy and the Challenge of Sustainability,* op. cit.

[108] United Nations, *Report of the Secretary General on We the Children: End-Decade Review of the Follow-up to the World Summit for Children,* op. cit.

[109] United Nations Secretariat of the Convention to Combat Desertification (UNCCD): http://www.unccd.int/main.php

[110] Food and Agriculture Organization, *Food, Security and Nutrition,* World Food Summit, FAO, 1996 cited in UNEP, *Global Environment Outlook 2000,* op. cit.

[111] United Nations Environment Programme, *Global Environment Outlook 2000,* op. cit.

[112] Ibid.

[113] Economic and Social Council of the United Nations, *Health and Sustainable Development: Report of the Secretary General to the Commission on Sustainable Development,* op. cit.

[114] United Nations, *Report of the Secretary General on We the Children: End-Decade Review of Follow-up to the World Summit for Children,* op. cit.

[115] United Nations Environment Programme, *Global Environment Outlook 2000,* op. cit.

[116] World Health Organization, *Strengthening Interventions to Reduce Helminth Infections: As an Entry Point for the Development of Health-Promoting Schools,* op. cit.

[117] World Health Organization, *Childhood nutrition and progress in implementing the International Code of Marketing of Breast-milk Substitutes*, EB109/11, 2001.

[118] Bateman, Massee, *The Unfinished Agenda: Microbiological Contaminants and the Burden of Disease*, Presentation at a children's environmental health panel discussion during the Second Session of the Preparatory Committee for the United Nations General Assembly Special Session on Children, February 2001.

[119] World Health Organization, *Strengthening Interventions to Reduce Helminth Infections: As an Entry Point for the development of Health-Promoting Schools*, 1979b, op. cit.

[120] Ibid.

[121] Talukder, Aminuzzaman et al., "Increasing the production and consumption of vitamin A-rich fruits and vegetables: Lessons learned in taking the Bangladesh homestead gardening programme to a national scale," *Food and Nutrition Bulletin*, Vol.21, No.2., United Nations University, Tokyo, 2000.

[122] United Nations (Department for Economic and Social Affairs), Promotion of Horti-Forestry for Sustainable Livelihood, *Sustainable Development Success Stories*, 2000.

www.un.org/esa/sustdev/success/SARD-22.htm

[123] United Nations (Department for Economic and Social Affairs), "Unlimited Responsibility of the Union of Indian Communities of the Isthmus Region," *Sustainable Development Success Stories*, 2000. www.un.org/esa/sustdev/success/SARD-8.htm.

Chapter 4: Global Environmental Problems

[1] Intergovernmental Panel on Climate Change (IPCC), Climate Change 2001: The Scientific Basis – *Third Assessment Report*, IPCC, Geneva, 2001.

[2] Ibid.

[3] Ibid.

[4] Intergovernmental Panel on Climate Change, *Summary for Policymakers: Climate Change 2001: Impacts, Adaptation, and Vulnerability*, A Report of Working Group II of IPCC, Geneva, 2001.

[5] Intergovernmental Panel on Climate Change, *Summary for Policy Makers: Climate Change 2001: Impacts, Adaptations, and Vulnerability*, op. cit.

[6] United Nations Environment Programme, Ozone Secretariat: http://www.unep.org/ozone/

[7] United States Environmental Protection Agency, Children's Environmental Health Yearbook, EPA, Washington D.C., 1998. http://www.epa.gov/children/whatwe/ochpyearbook.pdf

[8] United Nations Secretariat of the Convention to Combat Desertification (UNCCD): http://www.unccd.int/main.php

[9] Ibid.

[10] United Nations Secretariat of the Convention on Biological Diversity (CBD): http://www.biodiv.org

[11] United Nations Environment Programme, *Global Environment Outlook 2000*, op. cit..

[12] Murray, C.J.L. & A. D. Lopez (eds.), *The global burden of disease: a comprehensive assessment of mortality an d disability from diseases, injuries and risk factors in 1990 and projected to 2020*, Harvard School of Public Health on behalf of World Health Organization and the World Bank, Harvard University Press, 1996.

[13] United Nations Children's Fund, *The State of the World's Children 2001*, op. cit.

Abbreviations

Terminology

ARI: acute respiratory infections
CFC: chlorofluorocarbons
DDT: dichlorodiphenyltrichloroethane – a chlorinated organic insecticide that persists for a longtime in the environment. It is disastrously toxic to birds, and is thought to cause cancer in humans.
DHF: dengue hemorrhagic fever
FRESH: Focusing Resources on Effective School Health
JE: Japanese encephalitis
ODS: ozone depleting substances
PAH: polycyclic aromatic hydrocarbons
PCBs: Polychlorinated biphenyls. A group of organic compounds that persist in the environment for long periods of time, and are known as bioaccumulants.
PM10: Small particles of diameter less than 10 microns
POPs: persistent organic pollutants
PVC: polyvinyl chloride. A type of plastic.
SSHE: School Sanitation and Hygiene Education

Organizations / bodies

CEHN: Children's Environmental Health Network
ECOSOC: United Nations Economic and Social Council
FAO: United Nations Food and Agriculture Organization
IPCC: Intergovernmental Panel on Climate Change
IPF: Intergovernmental Panel on Forests
NRDC: Natural Resources Defense Council
UCIRI: Union of Indian Communities of the Isthmus Region
UNAIDS: The joint United Nations Programme on HIV/AIDS
UNCBD: United Nations Convention in Biological Diversity
UNCED: United Nations Conference on Environment and Development (also known as "The Earth Summit")
UNCHS United Nations Centre for Human Settlements (Habitat) [now called UN Human Settlements Programme (UN-Habitat)]
UNEP: United Nations Environment Programme
UNESCO: United Nations Educational, Scientific and Cultural Organization
UNFCCC: United Nations Framework Convention on Climate Change
UNFF: United Nations Forum on Forests
UNICEF: United Nations Children's Fund
UN/CCD: United Nations Convention to Combat Desertification
USEPA: United States Environmental Protection Agency
WHO: World Health Organization
WMO: World Meteorological Organization
WRI: World Resources Institute

INDEX

Photo Credits

Cover photos (clockwise from top-left: 1) UNEP/Topham, 2) UNICEF/HQ97-0777/ Roger Lemoyne, 3) WHO/archive, 4) WHO/archive, 5) UNICEF / Nancy McGirr
6) UNEP/ Aimen Al-Sayyad
v: UNEP / Topham 0014507 / Wihan Kwandee
vi: UNICEF / HQ99-0301/ Giacomo Pirozzi
4: UNICEF/HQ93-0501/ Cindy Andrew
13: UNICEF / HQ01-0160 / Giacomo Pirozzi
16: UNICEF / HQ97-0998 / Jeremy Horner
27: UNICEF / DOI90-0027 / Ellen Tolmi
28: UNICEF / HQ94-0632 / Dora Gutierrez
35: UNICEF / HQ00-0910 / Roger Lemoyne
40: UNICEF / DOI93-1175 / Jeremy Horner
42: UNEP / Topham 0221845 / Scracity Nigeri
45: UNICEF/ HQ00-0578/ Shehzan Noorani
53: UNICEF / 91-0297 / Shinichi Asabe
68: UNEP / Topham 0146515 / Vladimir Akimov
77: UNEP /Topham 0020649 / Ivo Demi
85: UNEP /Topham 0022401
86: UNEP /Topham 0034195 / Kurt Adams
98: UNICEF / DOI95-0069 / Shadid
101: UNEP/ Topham 0199179 / Maria Teresa Diaz-Colocho
107: WHO / archive
116: UNICEF / HQ92-0491 / Nancy McGirr